0471793337   Cf

RADIATION SAFETY
Protection and Management for Homeland Security and Emergency Response

LARRY A. BURCHFIELD
President & Chief Executive Officer
Radiochemistry Society
Richland, Washington

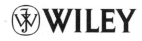
A JOHN WILEY & SONS, INC., PUBLICATION

Published by John Wiley & Sons, Inc., Hoboken, New Jersey
Published simultaneously in Canada

For general information on our other products and services or for technical support, please contact our Customer Care Department within the United States at (800) 762-2974, outside the United States at (317) 572-3993 or fax (317) 572-4002.

Wiley also publishes its books in a variety of electronic formats. Some content that appears in print may not be available in electronic formats. For more information about Wiley products, visit our web site at www.wiley.com.

Library of Congress Cataloging-in-Publication Data:

Burchfield, Larry A., 1951–
  Radiation safety: protection and management for homeland security and emergency response / Larry A. Burchfield.
     p.; cm.
  Includes bibliographical references and index.
  ISBN 978-0-471-79333-5 (cloth)
  1. Radiation injuries—Prevention. 2. Radiation—Safety measures. 3. Nuclear crisis control. 4. Nuclear terrorism. I. Title.
  [DNLM: 1. Radiation Injuries—prevention & control. 2. Nuclear Warfare—prevention & control. 3. Radiation Protection—methods. 4. Risk Assessment. 5. Safety Management. 6. Terrorism—prevention & control. WN 650 B947r 2009]
  RA569.B838 2009
  363.325'9—dc22
                                                                                    2009001781

Printed in the United States of America

10 9 8 7 6 5 4 3 2 1

Dedicated to My Father Jess N. Burchfield
in Honor of His 80th Birthday

CONTENTS

9   MEDICAL TREATMENT OF RADIOLOGICAL INJURIES   129

**10 CLEANUP AND DECONTAMINATION AFTER
A RADIOLOGICAL INCIDENT   141**

PREFACE

In reality, a significant amount of radioactive material and high levels of exposure are required to create a national or even a local health emergency. In practice, even small or suspected amounts of radiation are enough to cause mass panic and pandemonium.

Even before the introduction of the A-bomb in the 1940s, atomic radiation existed as a weapon of mass deception. Misinformation about mutant life forms; spies smuggling green, glowing orbs in their briefcases; and rumors of assured Armageddon swirled throughout society. Today's terror threats that involve radiological attacks, although rooted in reality, are similarly exaggerated, which makes them effective as weapons of fear and terrorism.

The truth about radiation lies somewhere between the terrifying and the mundane. We are surrounded by radiological sources every day: in our homes and industries, the food we eat, the medical care we receive, and even from the earth itself. Radiation makes our modern way of life possible. Yet, for most of the public it is shrouded in mystery. Take, for example, the 1979 accident at the Three Mile Island nuclear reactor. Although radiation levels in the area barely rose above normal, persistent public fear resulted in cases of long-term physiological stress and symptoms unrelated to radiation exposure.

A similar situation occurred in Lima, Peru, less than a year ago when a meteorite struck the region. Hundreds of local residence complained of dizziness, nausea, and headaches as a result of what they believed to be radiation poisoning suspected to be from the meteorite. However, nuclear physicists in the area ascertained that the meteorite's low level of radioactivity could in no way affect the population's health, and regional health directors agreed that none of the cases were attributable to the meteorite itself. They were all brought on by self-induced *fear* of radiation.

However, not all nuclear anxieties are unjustified. Very recently, hundreds of pages of blueprints for manufacturing advanced nuclear warheads and weapons-grade uranium were found encrypted in the computer files of a renowned black market smuggling ring. United Nations officials and International Atomic Energy Agency investigators believe these plans could have been copied extensively and sold off to rogue nations, terror cells, and nefarious regimes worldwide.

The designs found are for sophisticated, yet compact, nuclear warheads that could fit perfectly atop conventional ballistic missiles—exactly like the ones Iran was testing when the discovery was made.

Although 30,000 of the files were destroyed, some had already been sent to computer networks in Dubai, which was the center of the smuggling operation. Experts worry that copies of the blueprints are still circulating, although no one knows exactly where they are.

In these times when the fear of a large-scale radiological event exists alongside the technology to make it a reality, the best strategy we have is to educate ourselves about the facts of radiation and defend ourselves against the fiction.

FOREWORD

This resource is essential for those involved with planning and implementing homeland security and emergency response for a radiological disaster. This book provides an excellent guide to understanding the myriad details needed during a nuclear crisis.

Although the subject matter of radiation safety is highly complex, Dr. Burchfield has masterfully woven the numerous details into a highly understandable text. He starts with the bombings of Hiroshima and Nagasaki and the impact those events had on the world. Writers and film makers now had a new topic for involving fear into the public. Literally hundreds of movies cast radioactivity as an evil curse on humankind. This legacy led directly to the notion that nuclear fear has the potential of becoming the *Godzilla of all fears*—both figuratively and literally.

Case in point, the first chapter is devoted to an extensive history of the origins of public fear of radiation and the exploitation of this fear by the entertainment industry. The second chapter deals with terrorism and how terrorists will most likely exploit this fear. From fear to the mundane, perhaps the truth lies somewhere in between.

Appropriately, Dr. Burchfield takes the reader through the important subject of natural radioactivity at its most basic level. Natural radioactivity provides an important context in which to understand this controversial and complex subject. Workers in radiation safety will find the subject vitally important to understanding the existence, the decay modes, and the energy released from nuclear decay as well as the adverse health effects that can ensue.

The age-old adage that *people do not plan to fail they simply fail to plan* is certainly true and reverberates throughout this important resource. This book covers a large span of material to help all involved in a nuclear disaster understand the required efforts to respond to and recover from a radiological emergency. It provides wide-ranging detail to formulate action plans for all aspects of a radiological disaster from first response to site closure.

Such a document requires a true subject matter expert on the many facets of radiation and radioactivity. In my 35 years in the nuclear industry, I have never known a greater expert in this area than Dr. Burchfield, and I enthusiastically endorse this text as a must-have resource for all involved in homeland security and emergency response.

MICHAEL R. FOX, PHD

Nuclear Scientist

Member:
Radiochemistry Society
American Chemistry Society
American Nuclear Society
Health Physics Society

ACKNOWLEDGMENTS

I would like to thank the countless thousands of dedicated public servants that serve as first responders, police, fire and rescue, military, and medical personnel. It is their dedication to serve others that helps keep our communities safe. Special recognition must also go to the 343 brave firemen who lost their lives while attempting to save others during the 9/11 disaster. "Greater love hath no man than this, that a man lay down his life for his friends." John 15:13 KJV.

Special thanks to Doreen Michleski for her terrific job in editing this work and to Ben Burchfield for the wonderful job in graphics design.

I also would like to thank Melinda, Ben, and Bryce for their love, support, and encouragement. Furthermore, I would like to thank Mr. Tim Bivens for his dedication, integrity, and hard work in supporting me and the Radiochemistry Society during the preparation of this manuscript. Last but not least, I am most grateful to Mr. Bob Esposito for his encouragement and support of this project.

ACKNOWLEDGMENTS

CHAPTER 1

NUCLEAR FEAR—THE GODZILLA OF ALL FEARS

'A man cannot be too careful in the choice of his enemies'

—Oscar Wilde

In the early 1940s, nuclear technology in America was a burgeoning field rife with possibilities for potential weaponry to be put to use in World War II. The year 1942 saw the world's first nuclear reactor, which was fashioned from a crude pile of uranium and graphite out of which cadmium rods (able to absorb neutrons) protruded. This ambitious experiment—stacked on the floor of a squash court at the University of Chicago and surrounded by concrete walls—was inauspiciously referred to as Chicago Pile-1.

When the cadmium rods were removed from the pile, neutrons were released, which caused fission and the splitting of atoms—hence, the creation of the first *man-made*[1] nuclear reactor. In that same moment, something in the

---

[1]In 1956, P.K. Kuroda speculated that a *natural* assemblage of uranium could form a **natural nuclear reactor**. He went on to point out that if such an assembly did exist, it would have gone critical 1.9 billion years ago. A *"fossilized"* reactor was found by the French in Gabon, Africa, in 1972. Many scientists have studied this reactor site and concluded that it had operated 1.7 billion years ago. This was indeed the world's first nuclear reactor—and it occurred naturally.

Radiation Safety: Protection and Management for Homeland Security and Emergency Response. By L. A. Burchfield
Copyright © 2009 John Wiley & Sons, Inc.

world shifted imperceptibly: Nuclear energy had gone from being hypothetical formula to practical device and thereby a historical fact.

Those humble beginnings in the lower level of an amateur sports arena belied the significance of what had just occurred: The world's first man-made self-sustaining nuclear reactor had been developed, ushering with it the birth of a new, nuclear age.

The public's initial reaction to this achievement was subdued. After all, what kind of impact could splitting a few atoms have on anything?

Within 3 years, the government's wartime efforts with atomic weaponry had sufficiently answered that question. Defense measures based on the principles of nuclear fission had stepped up considerably and were being secretly shrouded under the mysterious workings of the Manhattan Project, which was led by director Robert J. Oppenheimer. The first atomic bomb was tested by the U.S. Army's Manhattan Engineer District in July of 1945 in the Alamogordo Desert, which is a remote region of New Mexico. After witnessing this atomic trial run (called the Trinity test), Oppenheimer famously quoted the Bhagavad Gita, an ancient Sanskrit text: "Now I am become death, the destroyer of worlds." Because of the high degree of secrecy, the American public, however, remained unaware of the potential for destruction that had been unleashed in the desert.

That is, until everything changed forever on August 6, 1945.

1.1   THE BOMBING OF HIROSHIMA AND NAGASAKI

President Truman's decision to drop an atomic bomb (nicknamed "Little Boy") on Hiroshima on August 6, 1945 and then to drop another ("Fat Man") 3 days later on Nagasaki brought World War II (WWII) to a decisive end, with Japan's surrender shortly thereafter on August 15, 1945.

Of course, many Americans rejoiced in the victory. The A-bomb brought to a swift close a battle that had been raging on for 6 years and threatened to continue indefinitely, draining both domestic resources and finances, and claiming the lives of what could have arguably been tens of thousands of additional Allied soldiers.

However, when Japan finally signed the surrender on September 2, 1945, U.S. troops were returning to a homeland dramatically different than the one they had left.

1.2   NUCLEAR FALLOUT IN AMERICA

Although the end of the war was obviously good news, newsreel images of the atomic aftermath and declassified films of mushroom clouds exploding in the desert had indelibly burned themselves onto the collective American conscious.

Reports came in that within seconds of the atomic blasts, a total of approximately 110,000 Japanese had been killed; within days, the number of dead had doubled to 220,000—most of those were civilians. Thousands more were disfigured or would die in years to come because of radiation exposure.

It was apparent that not only Oppenheimer, but also America itself, had become a destroyer of worlds.

Its knowledge and possession of nuclear weaponry obviously positioned the United States as number one in the global arms race. The deaths of so many civilians and the near-destruction of two developed cities was more than enough to prove the effectiveness of atomic power and to impress or intimidate political opponents around the world—but it was also enough to make the American people question the safety of their government's domestic nuclear experiments and the attendant radioactivity.

It also begged the question that still resonates today: What would happen if these weapons—or the plans with which to build them—were to fall into the wrong hands?

In the weeks after Japan's surrender, the post-war sense of euphoria and security with which many U.S. citizens regarded their country's international dominance and recently exhibited, seemingly impenetrable defense policy were short lived. The atmosphere started to disintegrate into one of shared uneasiness, a sort of American zeitgeist of anxiety, as thoughts of nuclear power gave way to nuclear paranoia.

1.3 WMDs: WITNESSES OF MASS DESTRUCTION

Media images compounded the problem of atomic anxiety. Newsreels and footage of the nuclear explosion tests carried out in the desert of New Mexico were declassified by the U.S. military and shown relentlessly in the U.S. media, partly as pure news reporting and partly as an attempt at patriotic propaganda. However, the effects of overexposure to that kind of previously unseen, man-made mass destruction had an unforeseen negative impact on the American psyche. One can relate it to the more recent images of the World Trade Center buildings collapsing on 9/11; studies have shown that even almost 7 years after the tragedy, viewers who see the familiar footage broadcast in an unexpected context still feel a sense of powerlessness and loss of control at not knowing when or where they will be exposed to these images. In that sense, the anxiety one feels about randomly having to "relive" those moments through the media mirrors the same fear of uncertainty about when and if another terrorist attack will occur.

Witnessing the explosion of atomic weapons on their own soil (albeit by their own government) left a lot of Americans shaken. The issue of exposure to radioactivity became a by-product of exposure to images of nuclear testing.

Although the sudden increase in visibility of the mushroom cloud images contributed to a national nuclear unease, invisibility also played a significant part. The American public, like the Japanese citizenry, had been kept largely in the dark about the advances in nuclear weaponry until it was already too late. The general lack of knowledge about all things nuclear on the part of the American public added to their mistrust: The government had kept the information hidden all too well, not only from the enemy but also from its own people. The questions were as follows: What have we been exposed to and what new era of warfare are we being dragged into? And the underlying worry was as follows: Are we psychologically and physically prepared?

In addition, the fact that atoms themselves are invisible lent a feeling of the supernatural (or supranatural) to nuclear fission. The seemingly arcane knowledge about atomic energy was regarded by most Americans as belonging exclusively to the realm of scientists and secret government agencies (unlike guns and grenades, these new weapons were even out of the hands of the soldiers themselves).

The concentrated amount of death and devastation contained in a single atomic bomb, although based on simple laws of physics, made it seem almost alien. Richard Rhodes, the author of *The Making of the Bomb* commented that Einstein's equation $E = mc^2$ had been demonstrated for the first time to the world, in a horrifying way, by dropping the bombs on Japan. This also had a sobering impact on world politics. As Rhodes points out, if one graphs the number of deaths caused by war, there was in mankind's history an exponential rise in the death toll at the end of WWII (estimated to be 47 million). After which there was a radical drop to perhaps one million per year for the rest of the 20th century. Clearly, the bomb had a dramatic impact on not only going to war but also on policymakers' opinions about the futility of war.

And this is where the entertainment industry enters the nuclear equation.

1.4 FEAR AND THE FILM INDUSTRY

Within weeks of the atomic bombing of Japan, Hollywood filmmakers rushed to edit the declassified footage of mushroom clouds and nuclear testing into their products: from noir spy thrillers and pseudo-documentaries to B-level (and further down the alphabet) science fiction movies. The already terrifying true-life images of A-bombs exploding were capitalized on by the film industry and spliced alongside what were considered, at the time, even more unimaginably terrifying images of mutant monsters, atomic-powered aliens, and nuclear arms-induced Armageddon.

One of the first films on the scene was Henry Hathaway's *The House on 92nd Street*, which was released a mere month and a half after the bombing of Hiroshima. Logistically, the movie must have already been in post-production at the time, but it is apparent that a few lines of dialog (no footage, however) were added before its release to allude to the new nuclear threat. Although the film is a straightforward spy thriller, the Nazi infiltrators living in New York City were given a more pointed, updated purpose than simply smuggling U.S. military plans out of the country: Their new goal was to find the unspecified "secret ingredient of the atomic bomb."

Although it is amazing to think of the speed at which the entertainment industry sought to exploit the cataclysmic turn of events, this is not to say that works of film or fiction about the potential threat of radium and nuclear fission did not exist before the dropping of the first atomic bomb. Some science fiction writers in the late 1930s and 1940s (such as H.G. Wells) had already described accounts of the world coming to an end because of molecular-level mishaps. A few even came so close to the clandestine information involved in the Manhattan Project that they were censored by the U.S. government.

Even 2 years before the advent of the A-bomb, as unlikely a source of political realism as Batman used a plot in which Asian enemies tried to get their hands on secret American stockpiles of radium. The undisclosed use of this radium by evil forces would pave the way for their plans of world domination.

Could it be that Batman had gotten it right all along?

According to Hollywood, yes. Its role as atomic aggressor had ironically turned America into the ultimate target—if only on film, for the time being.

1.5 CELLULOID SPIES

A slew of movies released in 1945 and the years (and decades) following depict the United States as a country crawling with spies intent on finding the "secret" atomic formula.

Perhaps the most iconic of atomic, apocalyptic endings was delivered in Robert Aldrich's famous example of film noir, *Kiss Me Deadly*. In this adaptation of Mickey Spillane's spy novel, the hero/anti-hero Mike Hammer unintentionally unleashes an atomic explosion that causes the end of the world when curiosity gets the better of him, and he opens a briefcase containing the "great whatsit" (radium?).

Throughout the film, enemy agents have been trying to kill him to take possession of the briefcase; yet, once it is safely delivered, Hammer himself (in a reprisal of the archetypical, unaffiliated American detective role seen so many times in film noir) is the one who unwittingly unleashes the atomic explosion and watches in the movie's final frames as the world is swallowed up in an enormous mushroom cloud. *Kiss Me Deadly* resonated so strongly with post-war American audiences because it captured the sense of both nihilism and naïveté with which most citizens approached the issue of nuclear weapons and nuclear energy.

1.6   ATOMIC NATURE RUN AMOK

Spies, however, are not the only things that celluloid America was crawling with. Science fiction films of the 1950s (reacting to the recent Soviet threat of atomic warfare) show the country being invaded by insects bent on destruction, having gained their enormous size and powers through inadvertent exposure to radiation. From giant ants (*Them!*) and spiders (*Tarantula*) to a human-hybrid fly formed during a laboratory accident (*The Fly*), these mutant creations of popular culture, when studied together, point to a larger, more serious national concern: What effects would atomic radiation have on the environment?

In on-screen representations, America was open to an atomic attack both from below (out of the depths of the ocean in *It Came From Beneath the Sea* and from the Earth's core in *The Beast From 20,000 Fathoms*) and above (from outer space in *The Day The Earth Stood Still*). The giant insects, mutant monsters and, atomically armed aliens were special effects-enhanced stand-ins for Americans' real concerns about what radiation could do (or had already done) to the water supply, soil, and air.

In addition to the Soviets' amped up Cold War weaponry, the reports of disfigurement, deformed babies, and radioactive fallout that had still plagued Japan 10 years after the bombings weighed heavily on our country's conscience, even in the form of our commercial entertainment.

In 1955, perhaps the most notorious example of post-atomic war anxiety was released: *Godzilla, King of the Monsters*. What makes this film and its subsequent series most notable is not only the way it was embraced by the American public but also the fact that it was produced in Japan and was later dubbed with the stand-in reporter Steve Martin played by Raymond Burr. This gave a mechanism through which the Japanese movie could become an "American" movie without the traditional dub-line. Burr reprised this same role almost 30 years later in *Godzilla* 1985.

Watching the mutant, atomically enhanced creature come forth from an ocean tainted by radioactive waste to wreak havoc on unsuspecting Japanese citizens instilled fear (perhaps mixed with remorse) in audiences across the United States.

Oddly, *Godzilla* seemed to underscore a common link that American and Japanese citizens shared: Both had atomic bombs exploded in their countries by the U.S. government. The "God" in the title, then, refers less to America in general as a superpower and more to the specific scientific and governmental agencies who controlled atomic power—and, thus, the fate of the world. The monster itself is metaphorical as that power having gone out of control and as the mutant (or at least genetically mutated) strains of life that radioactivity could engender.

The spy thrillers, science fiction films, dramas, and monster movies that were made immediately after the atomic bombing of Hiroshima and Nagasaki, that continued throughout the Cold War period, that focused on nuclear accidents throughout the 1970s and 1980s, and that still grip us with apocalyptic anxiety today show that the dread associated with atomic energy and the effects of radiation has never entirely abated. At most, like the mutant life forms featured in many of these films, it lays dormant, ready to resurface at any time.

1.7 POST-WAR NUCLEAR REACTIONS

Within a year of the atomic attack on Japan and its subsequent surrender, the United States' official stance on nuclear weaponry had shifted significantly.

Robert Oppenheimer, who had been called "the father of the atomic bomb," quit his work for the U.S. Department of Defense and became chief advisor of the U.S. Atomic Energy Commission, which had been recently established to turn national attention away from nuclear weaponry and toward the application of atomic energy for more peaceful, productive, nonwartime uses. (From that position, Oppenheimer would later speak out against the escalating nuclear arms race between the United States and the Soviet Union.)

In 1946, the U.S. military asked inhabitants of Bikini Atoll in the Marshall Islands (a territory America overtook from Japan during the war) to leave the area so it could be used for additional, nondomestic nuclear testing. Unlike the Trinity trials in New Mexico, which were focused on military defense, these new, overt rounds of testing were ostensibly intended to regulate safety as well as to ensure "the good of mankind and to end all world wars" (according to U.S. Armed Forces spokesman Commodore Ben H. Wyatt).

The Pentagon had already reported on the American military's urgent need for having bombed Hiroshima and Nagasaki, which indicated in its official documentary, *The Beginning of the End*? (released in 1946 through MGM), that the drastic move was necessary because the Japanese government[2] had been close to completion of its own nuclear weapon.

---

[2] A recent documentary produced by the History Channel titled *Japan's Atomic Bomb* validates this premise. Documents detailing Japan's efforts at building a nuclear weapon were smuggled out of the country in 1949 by a young scientist by the name of Paul K. Kuroda. It was the author's privilege to study under Professor Kuroda, at which time (circa 1984) these documents were revealed to the author.

In the meantime, Japan had already begun working on treaties against nuclear armament, which would culminate in the 1960s with its self-imposed Three Non-Nuclear Principles disavowing possession, production, and introduction of atomic weaponry.

It seemed that, for the time being, the radioactive genie had been shoved back inside its bottle.

1.8   THE SPECTER OF COLD WAR

The relative post-war peace that Americans seemed to have made with their newfound nuclear power eroded in an instant on August 29, 1949—the day the Soviet Union set off its first successful atomic bomb.

A few weeks later, news of the Soviets' atomic achievement reached American shores and sent shockwaves through a country already familiar with firsthand accounts of the effects of atomic radiation. Estimates by scientists and government officials had stated emphatically that it would be more than a decade before it would be possible for the Soviets to have the bomb. This erroneous assumption was based on another erroneous assumption—that nuclear secrets remain secret. This of course led many to believe that spies were to blame, which was true. This incident in history is only magnified today with the news that even small rogue nations have now garnered nuclear secrets. What is old becomes new and fashionable again even in the realm of nuclear secrets.

Although the U.S.S.R. had sided with the Allies during World War II, it was excluded from secret information about atomic weaponry that had been shared between British and American intelligence; thus, the already strained relations among the countries deteriorated almost immediately after the fighting had ended. The Western allies were wary of communism in general—and of Stalin specifically.

A stunned President Truman refused to accept that Russian scientists had, on their own, discovered the "secrets" of atomic fission (which had been hinted at by Einstein in his famous equation $E = mc^2$ almost four decades earlier and later applied by the Germans in late 1938)—especially so soon after the United States had. Instead, he publicly announced the presence of spies who were working in American intelligence.

This "official" presidential proclamation seemed to lend credence to the Red Scare suspicions that had been plaguing the U.S. administration—and the Hollywood film industry—since 1947. Although the House Committee on Un-American Activities (HUAC) had been in place since the 1930s to check on the propagation of subversive materials (particularly, at that time, anti-American or pro-Nazi messages, whether interpersonal or spread through the media), its focus had shifted after the end of World War II to almost exclusively sniffing out the dissemination of communist propaganda within the country.

Infamously, HUAC held a series of hearings to examine members of the entertainment industry on suspicion of being Soviet sympathizers. Producers, directors, and actors who had been making, either with express government commission or consent, pro-Russian films just a few years earlier, when the U.S.S.R. was siding with the Allied forces, were now coming under scrutiny as "reds" or, worse yet, Russian spies. For refusing to cooperate with Congress, certain workers within the industry were blacklisted and refused work, most notably the Hollywood Ten.

With Truman's proclamation about Soviet espionage (reaching a crescendo in the 1960s with the trial and execution of the Rosenbergs), the scrutiny under which average American citizens lived amid accusations of the "red menace" and the examples that HUAC was making of a select group of high-profile people—all in addition to the Russians' new atomic intelligence—another wave of paranoia swept the country.

Fear of a nuclear winter chilled most Americans to the core; thus, the Cold War began in earnest.

1.9 THE FEARFUL FIFTIES

By the early 1950s, the U.S. military had established permanent test sites for nuclear weapons in the Nevada desert and the Marshall Islands. By then, most of the American public was resigned to the fact that the only way to avoid an impending nuclear war with Russia was to accelerate the arms race; thus, newly developed hydrogen bombs were added to America's arsenal.

Amid government-sanctified anti-Communist propaganda films and individual members of Hollywood attempting to outdo one another in the production of patriotic, pro-democratic movies, America was once again awash in images of mad (Soviet) scientists intent on pushing a single red button to blow up the entire (free) world and undercover agents seeking to steal U.S. military secrets—both in movie theaters and on broadcast news media.

Unlike the spy thrillers of the late 1930s and 1940s, in which unspecified shadowy figures from Axis nations roamed the underground, the current crop of Hollywood offerings identified one single, unified enemy out to destroy us.

The constant threat of a possible Russian atomic missile attack on American soil is perhaps the most prolonged and persistent example of terrorism ever to affect our country.

1.10   DR. STRANGELOVE AND LEARNING TO LOVE THE BOMB

The U.S. government's policy of increased isolationism, as well as some influential politicians' well-publicized searches for Soviet infiltrators, stoked the public's panic about a potential outside attack.

At the same time, Russia's increased atomic strength ignited an almost contradictory belief among Americans that a strong military defense and arsenal were our best chances for avoiding nuclear apocalypse. A 1954 Gallup poll showed that 54% of Americans felt the H-bomb actually decreased the possibility of another world war.

Many historians argue that the change in U.S. administration brought with it a marked change in Americans' attitudes toward Cold War weaponry. Truman left office in 1953 to be succeeded by President Dwight D. Eisenhower; he was a decorated World War II veteran who was introduced to the American public as having played a major role in the defeat and disintegration of the Nazi Party. During the war, Eisenhower had acted as commanding general in the European Theater of Operations, and he was appointed afterward as the supreme commander of Allied Forces in the North African Theater of Operations and, finally, as general of the Army.

Whereas Truman's decision to deploy nuclear weapons on Japan seemed sudden (in that there was barely more than a month between the first nuclear tests and the actual bombing of Hiroshima, with no advance warning of either event given to the American public) and brought about a swift ending to the war, Eisenhower's policy toward the current Cold War crisis was that the country had best be prepared to remain in it for the long haul. The emphasis on nuclear weaponry had shifted from one of deployment to deterrent.

It was a change the American public could learn to live with.

In the years since the Cold War began, fears about the potential for nuclear war were subsumed into what soon became normal daily behavior: Students dove under desks during routine atomic air raid drills (this author remembers many such drills very vividly during his youth), and underground bomb shelters sprung up as quickly as aboveground swimming pools in suburban backyards. In a sense, the overall attitude of this time period, which was espoused by Eisenhower, was that the possession of nuclear arms became somewhat synonymous with the protection of the "American way of life." As long as the United States kept up its end of the arms race, the possibility of actual nuclear warfare was banished to a more distant corner of the American consciousness. This sentiment was later reaffirmed in the concept known as mutually assured destruction or "mad."

By 1957, U.S. citizens living in the Southwest had especially become so accustomed to the testing going on in Nevada (and so reassured by the government's declarations of health and public safety) that a new beauty pageant called Miss Atomic Bomb was created, and crowds from neighboring Las Vegas would set up beach chairs to watch nuclear "sunsets," cocktails in hand (see Fig. 1.1).

For perhaps the first time in history, long-held fears of nuclear annihilation sat squarely alongside an embrace of the benefits afforded by having (as opposed to utilizing) nuclear weaponry. Americans would continue to occupy this position uncomfortably for the next quarter-century.

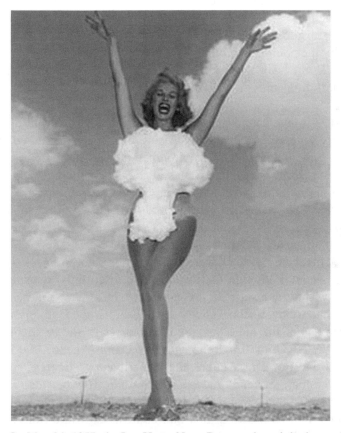

Figure 1.1. On May 24, 1957, the Las Vegas News Bureau released the last and, arguably, the most famous "Miss Atomic Bomb" photo of all to coincide with Operation Plumbbob at the Nevada Test Site. All Las Vegas Strip hotel showrooms had their own "lines" of showgirls, who performed in between the famous headlines. Don English took the famous Miss Atomic Bomb photo of Copa showgirl Lee Merlin at the Sands Hotel. With a cotton mushroom cloud added to the front of her swim suit, the publicity photo of the last Miss Atomic Bomb has appeared and continues to appear in hundreds of publications worldwide.

1.11 NUCLEAR TERROR REVISITED

Essentially, Americans' relationship to atomic energy has, since the discovery of nuclear fission, depended a great deal on the amount of information—and misinformation—divulged by both the government and the media (sometimes acting in accordance). This is true of almost any issue that, along with health implications, has ties to the country's military, economic, and political considerations.

However, a time comes when the public's fears runs head-on into facts about the safety of nuclear power.

That is what happened with the American public's perception of nuclear energy in the late 1970s and 1980s. Although anxiety over a nuclear holocaust never fully subsided after the initial outbreak of the Cold War, it was partially mollified by the country's economic and industrial booms in the latter half of the 1950s. In the 1960s, the U.S. military's involvement in a "hot" war in Vietnam left little energy and few resources to be wasted on Cold War concerns.

By the 1970s, nuclear power was being considered as a viable alternative to other energy sources, especially amid rising fuel prices, increased tensions in the Middle East, and heightened environmental awareness. In fact, 93 nuclear power plants across the United States all began operating within the same year, 1973, providing 20% of the country's electricity. Oppenheimer's long-held dreams of peaceful application for atomic energy were finally coming to fruition.

Until America suffered a meltdown.

In 1979, the Three Mile Island nuclear power plant in Pennsylvania overheated at its core. Although the meltdown released only a small amount of radioactivity into the surrounding area, no immediate injuries or deaths occurred. According to the U.S. Nuclear Regulatory Commission (NRC), detailed studies of the radiological consequences of the accident were conducted by the NRC, the Environmental Protection Agency, the Department of Health, Education and Welfare, the Department of Energy, and the State of Pennsylvania. Several independent studies were also conducted. Estimates are that the average dose to about 2 million people in the area was only about 1 millirem. To put this into context, exposure from a full set of chest X-rays is about 6 millirem compared with the natural radioactive background dose of about 100–125 millirem per year for this area. The collective dose to the community from the accident was very small. The maximum dose to a person at the nuclear site boundary would have been less than 100 millirems.

The real casualty of Three Mile Island was the "meltdown of public confidence" in the use of nuclear energy. Ironically, *The China Syndrome* (an acclaimed fictional film depicting the melting of the core of a nuclear reactor and the subsequent cover-up) was released on March 16, 1979—a mere 12 days before the accident at Three Mile Island. Hollywood benefited, and the country's use of nuclear power went into a tailspin (in terms of public confidence and in terms of a sharp rise in anti-nuclear sentiment). According to the U.S. Department of Energy, the last reactor built was the River Bend plant in March 1977. The last plant to begin commercial operations was the Watts Bar 1 plant in Tennessee, which came online in 1996.

Today nuclear power is making a "Nuclear Renaissance." According to the NRC, currently 23 applications are pending for 34 new nuclear power plants to be built within the next decade. This resurgence of confidence in nuclear has been brought about by high oil prices, lower cost of operation (nuclear is now the lowest cost per kilowatt-hour among the major energy production methods), no production of greenhouse gases, and an urgency for the United States to wean from the use of foreign oil.

After clashes between administrative policy and public opinion over the unpopular Vietnam War, many Americans' trust in the government had already begun to erode. The incident at Three Mile Island invoked further confusion, anger, and anxiety (especially coming less than two weeks after the release of *The China Syndrome*).

Old fears resurfaced: Even though nuclear power was now being put toward peaceful means, that did not mean it still could not harm us.

1.12 CHERNOBYL'S IMPACT ON CONTEMPORARY VIEWS OF NUCLEAR ENERGY

Seven years after the near-miss at Three Mile Island, an event occurred that would turn worldwide public opinion against nuclear power well into the next millennium: the explosion at the Chernobyl nuclear reactor in the northern Ukraine.

In April 1986, this accident released tons of radioactive material—400 times more than what was released by the combined atomic bombing of Hiroshima—into the atmosphere over three countries: more than 12 trillion international units of radioactivity in Becquerels (Bq) or disintegrations per second, most of which was released in the first 10 days. Close to five million people living in the surrounding vicinities were exposed to dangerous levels of radiation. In comparison, all the aboveground testing performed in the 1950s and 1960s is estimated to put some 100 to 1000 times more radioactive material into the atmosphere than the Chernobyl accident.

Less than 50 immediate deaths were attributed to the explosion; the effects were felt for years. A total of 237 occupationally exposed people were admitted to hospitals, and 134 were diagnosed with "acute radiation syndrome." Of these, 28 died within the first 3 months, whereas at least 14 additional patients died over the next 10 years; however, perhaps some deaths cannot be attributed entirely to radiation exposure. Two other people died in the explosion, and one more presumably died of heart failure. Additionally, some 200,000 people involved in the initial clean-up of the plant received average total body radiation doses of the order of 100 mSv (millisieverts). Ten mSv is equivalent to the dose of one general chest X-ray. Twenty mSv is also the dose limit currently permitted for workers in nuclear facilities. The average worldwide natural "background" radiation is about 2.4 mSv.

Within the group of 116,000 evacuated from the "exclusion zone," fewer than 10% received doses greater than 50 mSv; fewer than 5% received more than 100 mSv.

A sharp increase in thyroid cancer among children from the affected areas is the only major public health impact from radiation exposure documented to date. By the end of 1995, approximately 800 cases in children under 15 years of age had been diagnosed, mainly in the northern part of Ukraine and in Belarus. Three children died as a result of this cancer, which can be treated medically.

The only documented and attributed cancers are from thyroid cancer. This is because of the high levels of radioactive iodine that were released to the general population. No increases have been detected in either leukemia or malignancies other than thyroid carcinomas. However, a note of caution should be made that some effects may take years to show statistically significant levels of other types of cancers or other attributable radiation exposures.

Perhaps the greatest toll Chernobyl has had on human health has nothing to do with radioactivity. From this incident, numerous psychological health disorders, such as anxiety, depression, fatalistic attitudes, and other psychosomatic disorders, have been caused by mental distress. It is difficult, however, to separate these effects from those brought about by the collapse of the USSR.

Another important point to stress is that exact numbers related to the Chernobyl nuclear fallout are difficult to come by because the Soviet government stopped allowing radiation to be cited as the official cause on death certificates.

With the closing of the Chernobyl nuclear plant, the case for safe nuclear energy was indelibly damaged. Images of Chernobyl victims recalled the equally unsettling and terrifying photos taken of the atomic aftermath in Japan. The two separate incidents, although very different in nature, became inextricably linked in a lineage of nuclear terror that spanned decades and continents.

In America, President Reagan had already spoken out against the madness (the "mutually assured destruction") of maintaining nuclear armaments. Now, the explosion at Chernobyl was recognized as evidence of exposing the fallacy of "safe" nuclear energy.

As a result, Chernobyl and at its core, nuclear energy, has been framed by hundreds of Hollywood movies as a mutant monster that created mutated, deformed victims in its wake and that, in the minds of some, seems to elude human control.

1.13 THE MYTH OF THE LONE MADMAN

From the Axis forces that operated in World War II to the Soviet superpower during the Cold War, even to potentially sinister nuclear power plants that operated among us, Americans could always trace the sources of possible atomic threat, attack, or espionage.

That sense of certainty ended when our world fell apart on September 11, 2001. After 9/11, terrorism took on a whole new meaning. Our military began searching for terrorist activities in all corners of the globe. The fear of a nuclear bomb falling into the hands of an unhinged dictator or terrorist cell bent on destroying the Western world was the underlying basis for the American public's support of invading Iraq.

President Bush raised concerns by announcing that any extremist radical "able to produce, buy, or steal an amount of highly enriched uranium a little larger than a single softball" could produce a nuclear weapon within a year.

The myth of the lone madman is nothing new. Even before the first atomic bomb was dropped, films featured the iconic image of the mad scientist experimenting with radiation to one day realize his plans for world domination.

However, even regime leaders sympathetic to terrorist cells do not give away nuclear weapons or the materials with which to build them. For one thing, it costs too much. For another, it can be used against the very regime that provided it. After all, the first step toward world domination begins within a nation state.

Despite this logic, the terror caused by the possible possession of nuclear weapons by extremist factions or rogue nations has already taken hold of the American imagination and has held it hostage. Because the definition of a true terrorist lies in his ability to evoke and sustain fear, even the hint of a nuclear weapon has already done half the work for would-be terrorists.

1.14 FEAR OF AN UNKNOWN ATOM

Perhaps part of the strategy to relieve Americans' anxieties and negative reactions about all things nuclear should center around lifting the veil of secrecy that has enshrouded nuclear power for so long. Public acceptance is usually based on an increase in knowledge and information; in this case, that information includes how exactly nuclear fission functions, both the harmful and beneficial effects of radiation, what countermeasures are in place against atomic and radiological warfare, and the roles of medical personnel, the military, and first responders in radioactive scenarios. (All of these topics will be covered in the following chapters of this book.)

Since the Soviet Union has splintered and the Cold War arms race has ceased to exist, the perception of nuclear power as associated only with weaponry has also faded, taking with it much of the stigma surrounding its production.

As America looks to alternative fuel sources, nuclear energy is again at the forefront, for its "clean-burning" properties and low costs. In addition, the industry as a whole has one of the strongest safety records—with built-in security mechanisms as well as precise and exhaustive standards of regulation. Not one person in the United States has ever died as a result of a nuclear-related accident in the commercial nuclear realm. (Accidents are the anomaly, although of course they receive the most press coverage and therefore occupy a prominent place in the public consciousness.) With advancing designs for nuclear power plants, such as light water reactors, and an increasing reliance on computerization, the probability of accidents and human error has been greatly reduced.

Even though the potential for nuclear destruction is indeed real and has certainly been realized, it has also been exaggerated through decades of popular culture and public fear. Although more deaths over time have been attributed to auto accidents than to nuclear accidents or warfare, cars do not evoke nearly the same level of anxiety as nuclear reactors because we have accepted them as part of everyday life and find that their benefits outweigh the risks.

For nuclear energy to be viewed in the same light, it is important that the public be informed of its positive aspects. For example, nuclear energy reduces carbon dioxide emissions, which some believe contribute to global warming. The nuclear power produced in the United States today cuts the carbon dioxide being released into the atmosphere by an amount equivalent to taking 94 million cars out of commission. What this means is that nuclear power is perhaps more likely to save the Earth than to destroy it.

The key to nuclear safety has always been in the understanding of it, the harnessing of its use, and the implementation of maintenance and regulations. After all, nuclear energy is based on physical laws of nature; fear of atomic energy is a creation of mankind.

CHAPTER 2

TERRORISM AND NUCLEAR FIRE

But there shall be false prophets among the people, even as there shall be false teachers among you, who privily shall bring in damnable heresies, even denying the Lord that bought them, and bring upon themselves swift destruction. And many shall follow their pernicious ways; by reason of whom the way of truth shall be evil spoken of.

—2 Peter 2:1-2 KJV

While nothing is easier than to denounce the evildoer, nothing is more difficult than to understand him.

—Fyodor Mikhailovich Dostoevsky

2.1 A PROPHETIC WARNING

In 1999, 2 years before the 9/11 attacks, a Library of Congress study concluded the following:

Al-Qaeda's expected retaliation for the U.S. cruise missile attack against [its] training facilities in Afghanistan on August 20, 1998, could take several forms of terrorist attack in the nation's capital. Al-Qaeda could detonate a Chechen-type building-buster bomb at a federal building. Suicide bomber(s) belonging

Radiation Safety: Protection and Management for Homeland Security and Emergency Response. By L. A. Burchfield
Copyright © 2009 John Wiley & Sons, Inc.

to al-Qaeda's Martyrdom Battalion could *crash-land* an aircraft packed with high explosives (C-4 and semtex) into the Pentagon, the headquarters of the Central Intelligence Agency (CIA), or the White House. Ramzi Yousef had planned to do this against the CIA Headquarters. In addition, both al-Qaeda and Yousef were linked to a plot to assassinate President Clinton during his visit to the Philippines in early 1995. Following the August 1998 cruise missile attack, at least one Islamic religious leader called for Clinton's assassination, and another stated that 'the time is not far off' for when the White House will be *destroyed by a nuclear bomb.* A horrendous scenario consonant with al-Qaeda's mindset would be its *use of a nuclear suitcase bomb against any number of targets* in the nation's capital. Bin Laden allegedly has already purchased a number of nuclear suitcase bombs from the Chechen Mafia. Al-Qaeda's retaliation, however, is more likely to take the lower-risk form of bombing *one or more U.S. airliners with time-bombs.* Yousef was planning simultaneous bombings of eleven U.S. airliners prior to capture. *Whatever form an attack may take, bin Laden will most likely retaliate in a spectacular way for the cruise missile attack against his Afghan camp in August 1998.* [Emphasis added.]

These prophetic and sobering words were projected from the waning days of our last century into the opening days of the 21st century—and what is perhaps most disturbing about them is not what has already come true but what is still to come.

Many around the world are extremely—and justifiably—fearful about the use of a nuclear device by terrorists, which is the part of the "prophesy" that has not yet happened. The world still has not observed the use of nuclear "fire" as a weapon of terror; however, as history shows us, it could only be a matter of time.

This chapter delves into the general concept and background of terrorism and, from this perspective, will explore the disquieting notion of terrorists using the *nuclear option* and the potential *radiological disaster* that could ensue, engulfing our entire country—and the world—in the grips of nuclear terror.

Of course, the use of terror to target victims is as old as time itself—only the technology has changed.

2.2 HISTORY OF TERRORISM

In his book *A History of Terrorism*, Walter Laqueur declares, "Terrorism has long exercised a great fascination, especially at a safe distance, but it is not an easy topic for discussion and explanation. The fascination it exerts . . . and the difficulty of interpreting it have the same roots: its unexpected, shocking and outrageous character."

Perhaps one of the earliest cases of terrorism in the ancient world was the Zealots (the origin of the word "zealot") of Judea, whose religious fervor was so strong that they rebuked rule by Rome. They were labeled by the Romans as "ones with daggers," or sicarii, and were driven to assassinations of not only Romans but of other Jews who "collaborated with the enemy."[1]

Another terrorist group that has had an equal impact on our modern lexicon is the Assassins, who invented and honed the concept of terrorism as a political weapon between the 11th and 13th centuries. Murdering prominent officials or religious leaders was nothing new; however, ancient assassinations were most often isolated events that involved conspirators within the "inner circle." In contrast, the Assassins, who were located in what is contemporary northern Iran, used cunning stealth to execute their enemies repeatedly and systematically inside their own strongholds, thus gaining great notoriety. These incidents were used as propaganda weapons to bring about the fear and threat of imminent assassination, in this way turning political will in their favor, and new recruits were lured in by promises of paradise.[2]

---

[1]This "rebellion" became known as the First Jewish-Roman War, which is also called the Great Jewish Revolt. Their undermining of Roman authority became so open and widespread that eventually it led to the mass suicide of 936 Jewish rebels at Masada (meaning the "fortress"), which is a high mountain plateau that the Roman Legion X Fretensis had seized for more than a year in 72 A.D. In 2001, Masada was declared by UNESCO as a World Heritage site. Also, the head of the Israeli Defense Force, Moshe Dayan, initiated the practice of holding the swearing-in ceremony on top of Masada, which ends with "Masada shall not fall again."

[2]The Assassins were a splinter group of Shia Islam called the Nizari Ismails; in the early 11th century, al-Hassan became the head of the Ismailians, which was a rather obscure group of extremists who gained control of a rock fortress 10,000 ft above sea level called Alamut ("the eagle's lesson"), which is located in the mountainous region south of the Caspian Sea. From this vantage point, al-Hassan became known to the 11th-century Crusaders as the "Old Man of the Mountain" (which was added to our lexicon). Al-Hassan's tactics were perhaps made most famous by Marco Polo, who stated:

> "The Old Man kept at his court such boys of 12 years old as seemed to him destined to become courageous men. When the Old Man sent them into the garden in groups of four, ten or twenty, he gave them hashish to drink. They slept for three days, then they were carried sleeping into the garden where he had them awakened.
> "When these young men woke, and found themselves in the garden with all these marvelous things, they truly believed themselves to be in paradise. And these damsels were always with them in songs and great entertainments; they received everything they asked for, so that they would never have left that garden of their own will.
> "And when the Old Man wished to kill someone, he would take him and say: 'Go and do this thing. I do this because I want to make you return to paradise.' And the assassins go and perform the deed willingly" (from *The Adventures of Marco Polo*).

The exact origin of the word "assassin" (from the Arabic "hashassins," which means "hashish eaters" or "drug addicts") is in dispute because some scholars today believe that perhaps parts of Marco Polo's story are more legendary than historical, as a result of inconsistencies. However, Marco Polo did bring this remarkable story of the "Old Man" and his cult of Assassins to the West and he did actually visit Alamut in 1273 A.D.—nearly 20 years after the invasion by the Mongols (and a century and a half after the death of Al-Hassan).

The Assassins literally held the Muslim world in the grip of fear for centuries. Their leader (the "Old Man," as he was called by his murderous followers) directed campaigns of holy terror chiefly against his Turkish and Persian neighbors, and these fears were made real not through just some "ordinary" assassin but through clever disguises that the Assassins used, such as beggars, holy men on the street, or even trusted servants. Rulers, generals, and prime ministers could all be struck down at any moment. Assassins were even taught what to say in the event of capture and often times named innocent people as their conspirators to hide the true nature and extent of their terror organization.[3]

If some of this sounds familiar, it should. Although the Assassins no longer exist as a terrorist group today, the descendents of the sect live on in the millions of followers of the Agha Khan.

Why is this history relevant? Perhaps it is because this organization served as the model for modern archetypical Islamic terrorist groups—in some ways sharing striking similarities with Osama bin Laden's al-Qaeda.[4]

The history of terrorist groups clearly illustrates the depravity and deadly obstinence of atrocious evil and how it potentially threatens the entire civilized world, which demonstrates the kind of enemies that nations such as the United States face even today.

There can be no doubt that ancient terrorists have left an indelible mark on the 21st century in both word and deed. The only new twist to this equation is the potential for terrorists today to replace the "sicari" with the modern equivalent: nuclear weapons.

2.3   TERRORISM (UN)DEFINED

The modern English term "terror" dates back to the era known as the Reign of Terror (1793–1794) during the French Revolution, when it was used to describe the actions of the Jacobin Club in their rule of post-Revolutionary

---

[3]Threats sometimes had a more powerful impact than the assassinations alone. For example, a ruler might awaken with a dagger stuck in the pillow next to him, which usually was enough for him to succumb to extortion, bribery, or political favor. Perhaps the most famous of such events occurred with the great Saladin, who lived to tell of at least three such attacks and at times allegedly journeyed in an armored wooden cart for security.

In the end, it was not the Muslims who were able to purge this cancer of terrorism invoked by the Assassins. Instead, it was Hulagu Khan's Mongol hordes that eliminated them as a military force in Iran.

[4]It is dubious that any direct linkage (through culture or ethnicity) exists between the Assassins of old and al-Qaeda. However, various fundamental strategies of stealth coupled with assassinations remain unchanged. This theory is especially true when one considers the notion of their absolute conviction that "Paradise awaits those who kill in Allah's name."

France. At the time, "terrorist" had a connotation that one would take pride in, similar to being patriotic today. However, words and meanings do evolve.[5]

One of the last groups willing to use the word "terrorist" to describe itself was a Zionist organization called Lehi (Lohamei Herut Israel), which was known earlier as the Stern Gang. In 1946, these self-proclaimed terrorists killed 91 people to protest British rule. Most movements that resort to political violence and terror, however, prefer terms like "freedom fighters," "guerrillas," or "mujahedeen" (meaning "one who struggles")—and that includes al-Qaeda.

In recent years, the word "terrorism" has taken on politically charged meanings and uses. One's political, social, economic, and especially religious beliefs define who a terrorist is and is not. In short, very few other words in our modern lexicon define our view of "other" the way "terrorist" does, although terrorists can indeed be homegrown.[6]

In fact, no universal definition is available for "terrorism" because the meaning depends entirely on one's worldview and culture.[7] Some have claimed that the term is inherently pejorative and inflammatory; yet the old

---

[5]By the 1990s, people used the word "terrorism" to decry any attempts at intimidation or disruption. Hackers were referred to as "cyber terrorists"; Microsoft accused Apple of "patent terrorism" when it tried to monopolize intellectual property.

Even an antiterrorism bill passed by Congress defined the term so broadly that it could include anything from hijacking an airplane to breaking into government property or, as Geoffrey Nunberg, a scientist at Xerox PARC in Palo Alto, writes, "hitting the secretary of agriculture with a pie."

However, for today's press and most of the public, the word "terrorist" describes bomb-throwing or building-destroying madmen. By applying it mainly to radical groups, the term is acquiring a universal (or at least first-world) stigma.

Although most extremist groups called "terrorist" deny the accusation, they ironically continue to call their enemies "terrorists." This term as widely used in the West also reflects a bias towards the status quo. Violence by established governments is justified as "defense," even though some might consider that claim dubious. Attempts to oppose the established order is often labeled "terrorism," although this term would apply not only to many events in American history but also to all forms of colonization that involved violence against indigenous people and intentionally exposed them to diseases to which they had no immunity (for example, Jeffery Amherst's intentionally providing infected blankets to Native Americans, if true, could be described as one of the first examples of biological terrorism).

[6]The bioterrorism of 2001, in which anthrax spores were mailed to various U.S. media and government offices, was not, according to the Federal Bureau of Investigation (FBI), linked to the events of September 11. Instead, it was the work of a lone "homegrown" terrorist named Bruce E. Ivins. At age 62, Ivins had worked for the last 28 years at the government's elite biodefense research laboratories at Fort Detrick, MD. He had been informed of his impending prosecution—and subsequently followed this announcement by his apparent suicide.

[7]The *Oxford English Dictionary* defines terrorism as "a policy intended to strike with terror those against whom it is adopted; the employment of methods of intimidation; the fact of terrorizing or condition of being terrorized." *Webster's New International Dictionary* defines

adage that "one man's terrorist is another's freedom fighter" has also been espoused. What is a justifiable cause to one becomes an abomination to others.[8]

Twenty-first century terrorist activities involve assassinations, bombings, random killings, and hijackings; they are used for political, not for military, purposes and, most typically, by groups too weak to mount open assaults. Terrorism is a modern tool of the alienated, and its psychological impact is on the mass public.

Terrorism can, at least partially, be defined as the greatest possible degree of criminal activity, in which the largest populations can be affected and the greatest amount of economic activity disrupted—and nothing can achieve this on the world stage like nuclear weaponry.

---

terrorism as the "act of terrorizing, or state of being terrorized; specify: a) The system of the Reign of Terror, b) A mode of governing, or of opposing government, by intimidation, c) Any policy of intimidation."

The definition of the term in the *Oxford Concise Dictionary of Politics (2nd Edition)* begins: "Term with no agreement amongst government or academic analysts, but almost invariably used in a pejorative sense, most frequently to describe life-threatening actions perpetrated by politically motivated self-appointed sub-state groups."

Paul Wilkinson states the following: "In common with the authors of the American and Asian viewpoints, I bemoan the absence of a universally accepted definition of terrorism. The European Union has at last attempted to agree on a definition, though the result could hardly be described as a great success."

[8]Reuter's news agency prohibited the use of the word "terrorists" to describe those who pulled off the September 11 attacks on America. Stephen Jukes, who was Reuters' head of global news, explained: "Throughout this difficult time we have strictly adhered to our 150-year-old tradition of factual, unbiased reporting and upheld our long-standing policy against the use of emotive terms, including the words 'terrorist' or 'freedom fighter.' We do not characterize the subjects of news stories but instead report their actions, identity or background. As a global news organization, the world relies on our journalists to provide accurate accounts of events as they occur, wherever they occur, so that individuals, organizations and governments can make their own decisions based on the facts."

Naturally, Reuters' decision was met with concern by other news agencies. According to the *Christian Science Monitor*, "Reuters' approach doesn't sit well with some journalists, who say it amounts to self-censorship. They also argue that it's inaccurate. 'Journalism should be about telling the truth. And when you don't call this a terrorist attack, you're not telling the truth,' says Rich Noyes, director of media analysis at the conservative Media Research Center. 'A news organization's responsibility is to find the facts . . . not to play politics with its reporting.'"

As Rob Morse noted cynically in *The San Francisco Chronicle*, "News organizations are rethinking their use of the word 'terrorists.' The guys who flew planes into the World Trade Center and the Pentagon may be called 'alleged hijackers.' After all, you wouldn't want to prejudice jurors when the alleged hijackers come up for trial in hell."

2.4 LEGAL TAXONOMY OF TERRORISM

Although the concept of terrorism is controversial in its subjectivity, for terrorist acts to be legally charged as distinct crimes, "terrorism" itself has to be defined by laws and governmental agencies—and many have tried.[9] But as difficult as terrorism is to define both individually and legally, its focus is on actual damage to individuals and property and disruption of productivity, economy, and "normalcy," as well as an intention of intimidation. We will observe in the following chapters how nuclear technology in the wrong hands makes a radiological terrorist attack the most disconcerting and threatening; hence, both vigilance and preparedness are desperately needed.

---

[9]In 2005, a United Nations (U.N.) panel attempted to define terrorism as any act "intended to cause death or serious bodily harm to civilians or non-combatants with the purpose of intimidating a population or compelling a government or an international organization to do or abstain from doing any act."

The U.S. Federal Criminal Code (Chapter 113B of Part I of Title 18), better known as the Patriot Act, defines terrorism and lists the crimes associated with it as: ". . . activities that involve violent . . . or life-threatening acts . . . that are a violation of the criminal laws of the United States or of any State and . . . appear to be intended (i) to intimidate or coerce a civilian population; (ii) to influence the policy of a government by intimidation or coercion; or (iii) to affect the conduct of a government by mass destruction, assassination, or kidnapping; and . . . (if domestic) occur primarily within the territorial jurisdiction of the United States . . . (if international) occur primarily outside the territorial jurisdiction of the United States . . . " but against U.S. embassies, and so on.

Current U.S. National Security strategy has defined "terrorism" as "premeditated, politically motivated violence against innocents." The United States Department of Defense regards it as the "calculated use of unlawful violence to inculcate fear; intended to coerce or intimidate governments or societies in pursuit of goals that are generally political, religious, or ideological."

More pointedly, the U.S. National Counter-Terrorism Center (NCTC) describes a terrorist act as one that was "premeditated; perpetrated by a sub-national or clandestine agent; politically motivated, potentially including religious, philosophical, or culturally symbolic motivations; violent; and perpetrated against a noncombatant target."

Internationally, the British Terrorism Act of 2000 defines terrorism so as to include not only violent offenses against individuals and physical damage to property, but also those "designed seriously to interfere with or seriously to disrupt an electronic system" (which could involve shutting down a website whose views one opposes) as long as the act was "(a) designed to influence the government or to intimidate the public or a section of the public, AND (b) done for the purpose of advancing a political, religious or ideological cause."

The European Union uses a similar definition of terrorism for official purposes, which is set forth in Article 1 of the Framework Decision on Combating Terrorism (drafted in 2002). This article states that terrorist offenses are criminal acts against people and property, which "given their nature or context, may seriously damage a country or an international organization where committed with the aim of: seriously intimidating a population; or unduly compelling a government or international organization to perform or abstain from performing any act; or seriously destabilizing or destroying the fundamental political, constitutional, economic or social structures of a country or an international organization."

Terrorism is a crime and is defined by statute in many countries—and common principles among legal definitions of terrorism show an emerging international consensus as to meaning and an increased cooperation among law enforcement personnel in different countries.[10]

However, there are still disputes. Some regimes will not recognize the possibility of the legitimate use of violence by civilians against an invader in an occupied country, labeling all resistance as "terrorism." Almost all guerrilla groups (like the Chechen rebels) are accused of being terrorist, but almost all of them accuse the countries they are fighting against of being the true terrorists.

Others make a distinction between lawful and unlawful use of violence, despite political affiliations. It has been argued that the use of violence and weapons that deliberately target civilians and do not focus mainly on military or government targets is the fundamental basis of a terrorist act.

Although the use of violence for the achievement of political ends is shared among state and nonstate groups (and perhaps some may wish to include organizations such as the American Revolutionary Sons of Liberty, which are revered in American history), the difficulty is in agreeing on a way to determine whether the use of violence (who it is directed at and for what ends) is legitimate.[11]

Edward Peck, former U.S. chief of mission in Iraq, expressed the following:

> In 1985, when I was the Deputy Director of the Reagan White House Task Force on Terrorism, they asked us. . .to come up with a definition of terrorism that could be used throughout the government. We produced about six, and each and every case, they were rejected, because careful reading would indicate that our own country had been involved in some of those activities ... After the task force concluded its work, Congress got into it, and you can Google into U.S. Code Title 18, Section 2331, and read the U.S. definition of terrorism. And one of the terms, 'international terrorism,' means, 'activities that,' and I quote, 'appear to be intended to affect the conduct of a government by mass destruction, assassination or kidnapping.' Yes, well, certainly, you can think of a number of countries that have been involved in such activities. Ours is one of them. Israel is another. And so, the terrorist, of course, is in the eye of the beholder.

With so much uncertainty surrounding the very term "terrorism," one thing is for sure: The events of 9/11 confirmed that terrorism has attained a new

---

[10]In 1999, the U.N. Security Council unanimously called for better international cooperation in fighting terrorism and asked governments not to aid terrorists. The September 11, 2001, attacks by al-Qaeda on the World Trade Center and the Pentagon—which are the most devastating terrorist attacks in history—prompted calls by U.S. political leaders for a world war on terrorism, although the U.S. efforts to destroy al-Qaeda and overthrow the Afghani government that hosted it was initially unsuccessful.

[11]Geoffrey Nunberg commented, " 'Terrorism' is one of those terms like 'crusade,' which began its life at a particular historical moment—in the case of the crusades, in 1095 when Pope Urban II asked Europeans to wrest the Holy Land from the Muslims." With so many examples throughout history, can 9/11 really be thought of as the birth of "terrorism"?

status founded on suicide and mass murder on a scale that has changed life on the entire planet. Previous thinking provided a notion that "terrorists want a lot of people watching, not a lot of people dead." Suffice it to say that this has changed.[12]

Of course, the problem that terrorism poses is bigger than mere semantics. Terrorism is in part the reason for the war in Iraq. The U.S. government has not only spent hundreds of billions of dollars to counter groups that are elusive and difficult to characterize but also is having difficulty finding a resolute end to its "War on Terror." In fact, terrorism has become one of the biggest anxieties for Americans since 9/11, along with perennial concerns about the economy. But

---

[12]The proposed definition of "terrorism" by the United Nations in an address during the League of Nations Convention (1937) was: "All criminal acts directed against a State and intended or calculated to create a state of terror in the minds of particular persons or a group of persons or the general public."

However, in 1999, the language of the U.N. resolution had changed to include the following

1. A resolution that strongly condemns all acts, methods, and practices of terrorism as criminal and unjustifiable, wherever and by whosoever committed
2. A reiteration that criminal acts intended or calculated to provoke a state of terror in the general public, a group of persons, or particular persons for political purposes are in any circumstance unjustifiable, whatever the considerations of a political, philosophical, ideological, racial, ethnic, religious, or other nature that may be invoked to justify them.

A short legal definition proposed by A.P. Schmid to the United Nations Crime Branch (1992) proposed this formula: "Act of Terrorism = Peacetime Equivalent of War Crime." As the Academic Consensus Definition, Schmid submitted a somewhat longer version:

Terrorism is an anxiety-inspiring method of repeated violent action, employed by (semi-) clandestine individuals, groups or state actors, for idiosyncratic, criminal or political reasons, whereby—in contrast to assassination—the direct targets of violence are not the main targets. The immediate human victims of violence are generally chosen randomly (targets of opportunity) or selectively (representative or symbolic targets) from a target population, and serve as message generators. Threat- and violence-based communication processes between terrorist (organization), (imperiled) victims, and main targets are used to manipulate the main target (audience(s)), turning it into a target of terror, a target of demands, or a target of attention, depending on whether intimidation, coercion, or propaganda is primarily sought.

Thousands, if not hundreds of thousands, of diverse definitions of "terrorism" can also be found on the Web:

- The U.S. Department of Defense defines it as: "the unlawful use of—or threatened use of—force or violence against individuals or property to coerce or intimidate governments or societies, often to achieve political, religious, or ideological objectives."
- The FBI defines "terrorism" as: "the unlawful use of force or violence against persons or property to intimidate or coerce a government, the civilian population, or any segment thereof, in furtherance of political or social objectives."

not even the experts know exactly what terrorism is, let alone how to counter it completely. As Geoffrey Nunberg commented on National Public Radio's "Fresh Air" program and in his book *The Way We Talk Now*, "We are left like Supreme Court Justice Potter Stewart who, faced with the task of defining obscenity, simply said, 'I know it when I see it.'"

The thing is, after 9/11, we hope never again to witness terrorism on our soil again—especially a terror attack that involves the use of nuclear weapons.

Other organizations have this to say about "terrorism":

- "The systematic use of violence to achieve political ends is not new—among many other examples, it featured during The Troubles in Ireland before its independence in 1922. In recent decades, it has become a common tactic among a wide variety of groups, from independence movements to the secret services of various countries . . ."
- "Use of terror, especially the systematic use of terror by the government or other authority against particular persons or groups; a method of opposing a government internally or externally through the use of terror."
- "Any act including, but not limited to, the use of force or violence and/or threat thereof of any person or group(s) of persons whether acting alone or on behalf of, or in connection with, any organization(s) or government(s) committed for political, religions, ideological or similar purposes, including the intention to influence any government and/or to put the public or any section of the public in fear."
- "Systematic use of terror, manifesting itself in violence and intimidation. Terrorism has been used by groups wishing to coerce a government in order to achieve political or other objectives, and also by dictatorships or other autocratic governments in order to overcome opposition to their policies. Often anti-terrorist mercenaries will only do a job if they have carte blanche to do whatever they want . . ."
- "Acts of murder and destruction deliberately directed against civilians or military in non-military situations."
- "The systematic use of terror, the deliberate creation and exploitation of fear for bringing about political change."
- "A violent act in violation of the criminal laws of the United States, which is intended to intimidate or influence the policy of a government."
- "Terrorist activities are illegal and involve the use of coercion including the use of force, intended to intimidate or coerce, and committed in support of political or social objectives."
- "A psychological strategy of war for gaining political ends by deliberately creating a well-founded climate of fear among the civilian population. Such a strategy may be used by an occupying army on the occupied population. Many terrorist acts, especially against an occupying military or against illegal occupants, are acts of war or resistance, and not terrorism."
- "The calculated use of violence (or threat of violence) against civilians in order to attain goals that are political or religious or ideological in nature; this is done through intimidation or coercion or instilling fear."
- "'Terrorism' is a controversial and subjective term with multiple definitions. One definition means a violent action targeting civilians exclusively. Another definition is the

2.5 THE DEFINING PRINCIPLES OF TERRORISM

At no time in human history has terrorism played such a pivotal role. The reasons for this are diverse: We now live in a global community. Events that happen on one side of the world are immediately and instantly flashed to all parts of the globe. In the past, terrorist attacks were regionalized or subglobal. Such attacks (and there have been many) have availed themselves to localized regions and were minimized by the time it took the information to travel, gaining notoriety among only a localized population. Terrorist acts were locally suppressed, and in a subglobal climate, little or no effect was felt in other regions. The one factor that has changed all of this is indeed mass communications and the news media.

---

use or threatened use of violence for the purpose of creating fear in order to achieve a political, economic, religious, or ideological goal ..."

Even individual definitions vary:

- Brian Jenkins broadly states: "Terrorism is the use or threatened use of force designed to bring about political change."
- Walter Laqueur writes: "Terrorism constitutes the illegitimate use of force to achieve a political objective when innocent people are targeted."
- James M. Poland has said: "Terrorism is the premeditated, deliberate, systematic murder, mayhem, and threatening of the innocent to create fear and intimidation in order to gain a political or tactical advantage, usually to influence an audience."
- M. Cherif Bassiouni admits: " 'Terrorism' has never been defined ..."
- L. Ali Khan believes: "Terrorism sprouts from the existence of aggrieved groups."
- In 1989, Jack Gibbs attempted a more specific definition: "Terrorism is illegal violence or threatened violence directed against human or nonhuman objects, provided that it: (1) was undertaken or ordered with a view to altering or maintaining at least one putative norm in at least one particular territorial unit or population: (2) had secretive, furtive, and/or clandestine features that were expected by the participants to conceal their personal identity and/or their future location; (3) was not undertaken or ordered to further the permanent defense of some area; (4) was not conventional warfare and because of their concealed personal identity, concealment of their future location, their threats, and/ or their spatial mobility, the participants perceived themselves as less vulnerable to conventional military action; and (5) was perceived by the participants as contributing to the normative goal previously described ... by inculcating fear of violence in persons (perhaps an indefinite category of them) other than the immediate target of the actual or threatened violence and/or by publicizing some cause."
- Jason Burke, an expert in radical Islamic activity, summed it up as: "There are multiple ways of defining terrorism, and all are subjective. Most define terrorism as 'the use or threat of serious violence' to advance some kind of 'cause.' Some state clearly the kinds of group ('sub-national,' 'non-state') or cause (political, ideological, religious) to which they refer. Others merely rely on the instinct of most people when confronted with an act that involves

Terrorism, however, cannot exist without the right ingredients, just as fire needs oxygen, fuel, and a spark. The necessary "ingredients" for terrorism are nation states (individual countries), global media, and extremists.

2.6 NATION STATES: FUEL FOR NUCLEAR FIRE

Nation states (which is the specific language used by the United Nations) are often the targets or victims of terrorism; however, in some cases, they can be the facilitator and supporters. Either way, nation states are a necessary ingredient in terrorism. They are the "fuel" for the fire.

When nation states use military force against other nations, we refer to this as "war"; when extremists use military force against nations, we refer to this as "terrorism." Extremist groups often cannot be tied to one specific region of the world or country; their existence can be amorphous. Additionally, they may use or exploit nuclear technology from several countries, provide assembly of a nuclear weapon or material in a different country, deploy such a weapon from yet another region, and eventually target or blackmail an entirely separate nation. In short, terrorist groups today have the ability to cross borders across several nations simultaneously—and often with impunity.[13]

---

innocent civilians being killed or maimed by men armed with explosives, firearms or other weapons. None is satisfactory, and grave problems with the use of the term persist. Terrorism is after all, a tactic ... The term 'war on terrorism' is thus effectively nonsensical ... My preference is, on the whole, for the less loaded term 'militancy.' This is not an attempt to condone such actions, merely to analyze them in a clearer way."
- Robespierre called terror "an emanation of virtue; terror is nothing but justice, prompt, severe and inflexible." Shortly thereafter, as Nunberg noted, the "severe and inflexible justice of the guillotine severed 12,000 heads, including Robespierre's."

What all of this shows is that "terrorism," as a word and as a tactic, has led a double life for more than 150 years. The Russian revolutionaries who assassinated Czar Alexander II in 1881 used the term to describe themselves proudly. Even American author Jack London argued that terrorism was a powerful weapon in the hands of labor (although he warned against using it to harm innocent people).

[13]The concept of nation states (with precisely defined borders) is a relatively new phenomenon in mankind's history. In ancient times, sovereignty for various regions was controlled exclusively under "city-states"—that is, defenses, culture, and commerce were fashioned around a fortress or castle, which was later referred to as a "city-state." (Examples of ancient city-states include Rome, Babylon, Athens, Sparta, Thebes, and Corinth; lesser known ones include Chichen Itza and El Mirador as part of the Mayan civilization, and Smarkand, and Bukhara, which were located along the famous Silk Road. More modern city-states include Florence and Venice.)

As city-states grew and alliances were formed, they evolved into modern nations. A mere two centuries ago, empires and countries did not have well-defined borders; they were amorphous or loosely defined. It was only after the development of the science of navigation and surveying that clearly defined borders have come into existence. Rivers and other geological boundaries helped

However, war and threats of war are fueled by contrasting philosophies that exist across borders—and a very real by-product of this global friction is extremist groups, who exploit that discordance. They develop out of hatred and dissent and can result in contempt for any authority.

Many nations that nurture extremist groups do so as a diversionary tactic such as magicians use: misdirection. A specific brand of misdirection flies under the banner of *a false flag operation*, which is simply an action for which the perpetrator intends the blame (or credit) to be placed on a different party.[14] False flag terrorism includes terror by states, organizations, and agencies that is meant to be pinned on other factions to influence policy, public opinion, or military aggression without the actual source being discovered.[15]

So-called "state-sponsored terrorism," in which governments provide support or protection to terrorist groups that carry out proxy attacks against other countries, also complicates international efforts to end terror attacks and has caused many countries to place financial sanctions against nations that directly or indirectly support terrorists.

Political terrorism may also be part of a government campaign to eliminate the opposition (as under Hitler, Mussolini, Stalin, and others) or may be part of a revolutionary effort to overthrow a regime. Terrorist attacks are now also common tactics in guerrilla warfare. Governments find these difficult to

---

to define borders in the past; however, modern surveying and satellites have brought about much progress in precisely defining borders. Even recently, one heard the phrase "west of the Pecos" to describe a generalized region, and the Louisiana Purchase was defined by the watershed of the Mississippi River.

A nation's borders are also the point at which one nation's pride ends and another begins. Borders give a nation not only a sense of place but also a collective conscience, a sense of belonging, and a seat of culture and religion. Borders can be a point at which disputes erupt and wars begin. The recent events between Georgia and Russia are a perfect example. Borders disputes can also be used as an excuse for war, which, in fact, may be a better explanation for the troubles with these two former Soviet Union states.

A nation's borders can be its cradle for holding and developing culture and religion. Nations today are labeled as Christian, Jewish, Muslim, Buddhist, Shinto, and so on. A country's worldview and belief system can be shaped, for the most part, by the philosophy of a country's people. Open democracies tend to be open to the flow of ideas, whereas nondemocratic nations tend to dictate religious views and suppress alternate beliefs.

[14]The term originally comes from the naval concept of flying another country's flag to deceive and confuse other ships.

[15]History is filled with such examples. For instance, most scholars today believe that the Nazis torched the Reichstag in 1933 as a simple and blatant excuse to suspend democracy in Germany and as a means to install the dictatorial Nazi Party. In fact, Hitler immediately rushed to the fire and remarked: "You are now witnessing the beginning of a great epoch in German history ... This fire is the beginning."

prevent, although international agreements to tighten borders or return terrorists for trial may offer some deterrence.

What makes the fuel of nation states most flammable on the world stage today is when nuclear weapons are brought into the picture. Generally, nuclear materials are technically difficult to obtain with the resources and facilities established by a nation state. However, what is most disturbing in the 21st century is how the equation has changed with the very real possibility of terrorist groups arming themselves (through the aid of sympathetic nations) to exercise the "nuclear option."

The bottom line concerning nation states is that they will be facilitators for terrorist groups wishing to use the nuclear option, targets of the terrorists, or "bystander nations" (not immediately affected). The actual well-chosen target(s) for a nuclear terror attack will most likely be a major metropolitan city or cities (as was the case with 9/11), and the significant question on many minds today is as follows: Is there adequate preparation and cooperation among first responders, emergency medical staff, and interagency personnel to deal with and handle a radiological emergency or will mass panic rule the day? The jury is still out on this one.

2.7   GLOBAL MASS MEDIA: THE OXYGEN OF TERRORISM

If nation states are the "fuel" of terrorism, then the global mass media is the oxygen. Without oxygen, a fire cannot be sustained; similarly, without the global mass media, terrorism could not exist.

The "global mass media" is a recent phenomenon, having found its globalization through radio, television, and the Internet. Additionally, news outlets such as CNN, BBC, Sky News, ITN, PRI, Al Jazeera, and so on have succeeded in breaking through as "international" news media outlets. Together with the Internet, such organizations have unleashed a global news network.

In a worldwide economy, terrorism cannot exist without propaganda, the tool through which the *fear* of terror is propagated. Without induced fear, terrorism has little if any impact. To this end, terrorists must "get the word out" to cement their cause, promote recruiting efforts, and demonstrate their "power"—and news outlets are eager to report the story.[16]

---

[16]In his paper on "Media and Terrorism," Paul Wilkinson declares: "It would be foolish to deny that many modern terrorists and certain sections of the mass media can appear to become locked in a relationship of considerable mutual benefit. The former want to appear on primetime TV to obtain not only massive, possibly worldwide attention gains for them in the eyes of their own followers and sympathizers. For mass media organizations the coverage of terrorism, especially prolonged incidents such as hijackings and hostage situations, provide an endless source of sensational and visually compelling news stories capable of boosting audience/readership. . .once terrorist violence is underway the relationship between the terrorists and the mass media tends to become symbiotic."

A symbiotic relationship has thus developed between terrorist groups and global media in a manner that is both mutually dependent and complementary. In exploiting mass media, terrorist organizations have the following four main objectives:

1. To convey the propaganda of the deed and to create extreme fear among their target group
2. To mobilize wider support for their cause among the general population and international opinion by emphasizing such themes as the portrayal of themselves as "champions of oppression and the downtrodden," the righteousness of their cause, and the inevitability of their victory
3. To frustrate and disrupt the response of the government and security forces (for example, by suggesting that all their practical antiterrorist measures are inherently tyrannical and counterproductive)
4. To mobilize, incite, and boost their constituency of actual and potential supporters and in so doing to increase recruitment, raise funds, and inspire more attacks.

Terrorist acts create a media-rich atmosphere in which news organizations scramble to report the atrocities that are occurring. Media outlets are indeed first and foremost businesses: the more sensational the event, the higher the ratings. The higher the ratings, the more money a media organization makes.[17] Additionally, the media business is very competitive and often creates a "feeding frenzy."

Ultimately, it is the public's insatiable appetite for the "story" that can be claimed as the driving force, because even tragic accidents seem to draw the public like moths to a flame. In a free and open society, one that reveres freedom of the press and the capitalization and marketing of news, this begs the question: How does a responsible news organization balance the "need to know" without being used as a propaganda arm for some terrorist group?

2.8 EXTREMISTS GROUPS: THE SPARK THAT IGNITES TERRORISM

Fire needs fuel, oxygen, and an ignition source. In a similar manner, our global village contains all the necessary ingredients for terrorism to be ignited practically anywhere in the world.

---

[17]The market share of the audience provides a measure for increased revenues from advertisers. For example, during the 1979 Iranian hostage crisis, all the U.S. TV networks achieved an 18% increase in audience rating. According to Hamid Mowlana, the networks increased revenues by $30 million (in 1979 monetary rates) for each percentage point of audience rating.

During the 20th century, extremist organizations espousing different political and religious agendas have evolved in various regions of the globe. The good news is that the peak decades for the formation of extremist groups were the 1970s and 1980s. Since then, the rate of extremist group formation has dwindled considerably.

During that time, the political goals of extremist groups consisted of a diverse mixture of nationalist, left-wing revolutionary, right-wing radical, and religious agendas. The 1990s, however, observed the emergence of new extremist groups that mainly reflected religious fanaticism—and Islamic groups top this list.

Terrorism by radicals (of both the left and right) and by nationalists became widespread after World War II. Since the late 20th century, acts of terrorism have been associated with the Italian Red Brigades, the Irish Republican Army, the Palestine Liberation Organization, Peru's Shining Path, Sri Lanka's Liberation Tigers of Tamil Eelam, the Weathermen, and some members of U.S. militia organizations, among many others.

Religiously inspired terrorism has been linked to extremist Muslims associated with Hamas, Osama bin Laden's al-Qaeda, extremist Sikhs in India, and Japan's Aum Shinrikyo, who released nerve gas in Tokyo's subway system in 1995.

Despite the plurality of the meaning, however, many Westerners in general (and Americans in particular) are beginning to associate the term "terrorist" with those connected to the Muslim religion or a specific sect of Islam. This opinion is reinforced by some recent acts of terrorism attributed to Muslim groups, who have indeed claimed responsibility, as well as a lack of spoken condemnation against these acts by most of the Muslim world (although that may have more to do with fear of retribution than support).

In 2006, the National Counterterrorism Center of the United States gathered statistics indicating that approximately one fourth of all terrorist fatalities worldwide were perpetrated by "Islamic extremists." Specifically, these attacks took the form of airline hijackings, beheadings, kidnappings, assassinations, roadside bombings, suicide bombings, and rapes (the most infamous attack being the events of 9/11). Other notorious attacks, however, have occurred in Iraq, Afghanistan, India, Israel, Britain, Spain, France, Russia, and China.

Fewer Christians, Hindus, or Sikhs are connected with the term "terrorist" in the public vernacular—although representatives of each religion have been involved in terrorist activities both recently and throughout history. It is important to remember that terrorists from any group or organization, even acting individually, are equally dangerous, and governments, police, and military forces must investigate any potential terrorist planning, no matter the religion, background, or political connection of those involved.

Terrorism is not a singular movement but is a tactic used by a wide variety of groups, some of which are regarded and supported as freedom fighters in various countries or by various peoples. This "support" raises the specter of biological, chemical, and nuclear terrorism, and it reveals the complexity of dealing with—and defining—terrorist attacks. However, the following salient concepts must be considered in identifying terrorism:

1. Virtually no organization openly calls itself "terrorist."
2. Terrorist groups are generally amorphous with ties and cells that cross international boundaries.
3. Terrorism is a tactic, not an ideal of political or religious belief.
4. Terrorism is an unlawful act usually perpetrated across international boundaries with the intent to frighten, intimidate, or destroy.
5. Terrorism is often deployed under asymmetrical circumstances of manpower, resources, strength, and weaponry. In other words, terrorist tactics are an admission of being in a weak position politically, militarily, materially, or even philosophically.
6. Terrorism involves a tactical plan to maximize a climate of fear with a minimum reduction of resources and force structure.
7. Terrorism specifically targets innocent civilians and highly visible landmarks or shrines.
8. The goal of terrorism is to inflict fear to a wide audience through intimidation and disruption of governments and government services.
9. Terrorism is secretive and clandestine in nature and is fueled through money laundering and illicit activities, such as drugs, prostitution, theft, robbery, and so on. In short, terrorists believe that the end always justifies the means and therefore have little or no moral compunction.
10. Terrorist groups are cavalier and foster the "black and white" notion that only their "cause" is just, which leaves them inept and incapable of tolerance for opposing views, and usually doomed for extinction.
11. Terrorist groups use violence or the threat of violence to coerce governments, groups, or individuals into their demands.
12. Terrorist organizations generally present a false front of their illicit activities to their financial backers and state sponsors. Additionally, supporters and state sponsors are often willing to "turn a blind eye" and cling to a "righteous" indignation, which fuels and facilitates a fanatical cause.
13. Terrorism exploits young, idealistic followers by using the "romantic notion" that self-sacrifice is a path to a "higher regard and reward" for the recruit and "buy-in" by their immediate families.

14. Terrorist organizations and state sponsors make public acts of reward to family members of those "martyred." This is then exploited to entice recruits to help the families of "martyrs." In other words, emotion is a clever tool used to manipulate the naïve.

15. Terrorist organizations recruit scientists, engineers, and other professionals not only to enhance their organizational status but also to build and deploy weapons of fear and mass destruction. It is indeed a myth to think that terrorists are uneducated. In fact, most top leaders are usually very well educated. (Education, however, is not a likely quality of low-ranking, expendable recruits.)

16. Rarely does terrorism topple a government state.

17. Terrorist organizations exploit the news media to maximize propaganda.

18. Terrorist groups are deluded into a flawed thinking that their acts of violence and intimidation will create a total capitulation, surrender of will, and acceptance of the terrorists' agenda.

Conversely, it would be a mistake to underestimate the effectiveness of terrorist organizations the following reasons:

1. Terrorist groups have a high level of tenacity and resolve to disrupt lives, culture, and government services.

2. They can cleverly outwit the safeguards and security in place to thwart terrorist activity.

3. Their ability to endure hardship and harsh conditions is phenomenal.

4. They "market the cause" with zeal and charisma.

5. Terrorists' low-ranking recruits are often persuaded, then brainwashed, and ultimately exploited to commit suicide or other acts of horror most often against innocent and unsuspecting victims.

6. Diplomatic channels and state sponsors are often exploited to funnel people, information, and money, or to gather and pass intelligence.

7. Diffuse cultures and societies are melded into one mindset and purpose.

8. Many weaknesses of an open and democratic society are pinpointed and exploited.

9. Often they move with impunity across international borders.

10. Their scientific and technical capabilities (at a senior command level) for the deployment of weapons of mass destruction can be masterful.

11. Terrorists have the ability to operate through isolated cells and to communicate through sophisticated and clandestine means.

12. Their major "marketing" efforts rely on their ability to exploit the global news media.

So even though the number of extremist organizations may have dwindled, their support (both from government structures and the public sector) and fanaticism have not—and their messages can now be delivered through mass destruction.

2.9 NUCLEAR TERRORISM: THE ULTIMATE NIGHTMARE

The ingredients for a fire of terrorism are already in place, which could potentially trigger the worst terrorist attack mankind has known.

According to the International Atomic Energy Agency (IAEA), radioactive materials needed to build a nuclear device can be found in almost any country in the world, and more than 100 countries may have inadequate control and monitoring programs necessary to prevent or even detect the theft of these materials.[18]

When the nuclear "fire" does engulf us, what type of material will be involved? When and where will it be used? Who will deploy it? What type of "nuclear nightmare" will it result in? Answers to these questions are extremely difficult to pinpoint—although they are by no means hypothetical. Terrorist attacks using "nuclear fire" have the potential to create mass panic and large-scale confusion based on our collective—and easily ignitable— nuclear fear.

Adding to the complexity is the fact that few government officials, law enforcement agencies, first responders, and medical emergency staff are well trained in nuclear concepts, nuclear detection, or how to handle nuclear materials effectively and efficiently.

What is crystal clear, however, is that history, coupled with recent intelligence, has demonstrated that the world is not ready for nuclear terrorism— which makes it a perfect time for terrorists to strike the match.

---

[18] According to the Associated Press and CBS News (December 18, 2001), federal officials have admitted that Osama bin Laden has tried several times since at least 1992 to obtain components of nuclear weapons. In October 2001, he was quoted in a Pakistani newspaper as saying, "We have the weapons as a deterrent." Furthermore, documents seized in terrorist safe houses in Afghanistan yielded instructions on how to make various nuclear devices.

CHAPTER 3

RADIATION AND RADIOACTIVITY CONCEPTS

Many people associate the word "radioactive" with an eerie, green glow and "covert" clean-up by workers hidden inside Hazmat suits. It is an image long perpetuated by science fiction films, and it is exactly that: fiction.

Scientific fact, however, shows that we are surrounded by radiation in our daily lives. In fact, we would not be able to live the way we do in contemporary society without it. If you are inside now, there is a 20% chance that the light under which you are reading this book gets its electricity powered by a nuclear energy plant. If you are reading this in France (the country at the forefront of nuclear usage), that probability quadruples. To give you just a small idea of how radiation impacts our everyday lives, consider that the saline solution for your contacts has been irradiated to reduce the possibility of eye infections; many fruits and vegetables in your refrigerator were most likely exposed to radiation to kill bacteria and parasites, and the food in your freezer was treated with radiation as part of the sterilization process before packaging. And that is without yet having stepped out your front door!

Outside, instruments that use radioactive materials gauge road density; the airline industry uses radioactive substances to check for mechanical flaws in the engines of planes flying overhead. That does not even begin to take into account the naturally occurring radiation that has existed all around us in the

Radiation Safety: Protection and Management for Homeland Security and Emergency Response. By L. A. Burchfield

environment in detectable amounts for over five billion years, since the Earth was formed.

As shown by the domestic examples of radiation used above, certain levels are not only safe, they actually cause us to be safer in everyday life. We are also becoming increasingly dependent on man-made radiation in a variety of other fields, which allows us to enter a new age of medical, technological, and industrial achievements. Therefore, it is important that we increase our understanding of the concept of radioactivity and how it functions to dispel prevailing myths and distinguish between the amounts and types that are harmful or helpful to humanity.

3.1 WHAT, EXACTLY, IS RADIATION?

All matter is composed of elements that can be broken down into atoms, which are the smallest entities at which these elements retain their identity. Atoms are made up of three parts: protons (which have a positive electric charge), electrons (which have a negative electric charge), and neutrons (which have no electric charge at all and are therefore neutral). The protons and neutrons form an atom's nucleus, around which the electrons "orbit."

Some types of atoms (nuclei) are stable, which means that the number of protons and neutrons in the nucleus do not change over time. Atoms of the same element all have the same number of protons; however, some atoms of a particular element contain more or less neutrons than others. These atoms (with the same number of protons but different numbers of neutrons) are called isotopes. The word "isotope" is a Greek term coined by Margret Todd and Fredrick Soddy (in 1913) meaning at the same place—which implies that at the same place in the periodic table, one can have the same number of protons but a different number of neutrons. Some isotopes are stable, and some isotopes are radioactive and attempt to regulate or become stable by ejecting particles from the nucleus to achieve a stable nuclear state (in a process called radioactive decay). In general, nuclear decay produces a particle being emitted from the nucleus with high amounts of energy. Many types of particles can be emitted; however, the most predominant particles are alpha and beta particles. The alpha particle is composed of two protons and two neutrons. This particle carries a charge of +2 and has the ability to do great harm if its energy is released inside the body. On a relative scale, the amount of energy released by alpha decay is approximately 2,000,000 to 6,000,000 times more energetic than an ordinary chemical reaction (ordinary chemical energy often used by the cells in the body). It is the +2 charge and the high energy that causes the alpha particle to be so damaging to cells within the body. Within the body, a single alpha particle has the ability to kill three or four cells. However, an alpha particle that is emitted outside the body can be stopped with a piece of paper or even the first layers of skin. The bottom line is that alpha particles have the highest propensity to do harm inside the body; however, they pose no harm at all outside the body.

Beta particles are energetic electrons emitted from the nucleus. Beta particles carry a −1 charge and are 7344 times less massive than an alpha particle. This small mass of the beta particles causes much less damage to cells in the body. On a relative scale, beta particles possess energies of approximately 5000 to 2,000,000 times more energy than an ordinary chemical reaction. It is this diversity of energy and lack of mass that makes the beta particle less damaging to cells than alpha particles. Beta particles can be stopped by thick plastic or metals. If beta-emitting radioactive isotopes (radioactive isotopes are referred to as a radionuclides) are kept outside the human body, their harm will be greatly curtailed or completely stopped with either distance or shielding vis-à-vis materials, such as metals or plastics that are a few inches thick.

Another significant type of nuclear decay that could be of potential harm to humans is gamma ray emission. Gamma rays are a form of the electromagnetic spectrum that originates from the nucleus. Most gamma rays possess more energy than X-rays and therefore are more penetrating in general than X-rays. Additionally, most beta-emitting nuclides are also gamma emitters. Gamma rays have the same properties as visible light; however, they possess much more energy than visible light. All forms of light travels at 186,000 miles per second (in a vacuum) and so do gamma rays (the physicists call this form of radiation electromagnetic radiation). Gamma radiation is the most penetrating, and thick massive shielding is required to stop it. Gamma rays possess approximately 10,000 to 10,000,000 times more energy than an ordinary chemical reaction. Although gamma rays cannot be easily stopped, it is this simple propensity that makes them the least interactive with the human body. Gamma rays possess a double-edged sword—they are the most penetrating and can do damage from outside the human body (unlike alpha or beta particles). However, gamma radiation will most likely do the least damage because it is the least ionizing type of radiation (compared with alpha and beta). One other point about gamma radiation is that it is the easiest type of radiation to detect, and it can be detected the greatest distance from the source. Additionally, the intensity of gamma rays diminishes by the square of the distance, which means the intensity will be reduced by a factor of 4 by moving a factor of 2 away from any gamma source (moving a factor of 4 away from the source will reduce the intensity a factor of 16; and so on . . .).

The process to form stable isotopes usually liberates lots of energy—and it is that energy liberation along with released particles that is referred to as radiation. Radiation can be subdivided into ionizing and nonionizing radiation. It is important to understand also that ionizing radiation does not do harm unless these ionizing events occur inside the body. Therefore, blocking or stopping ionizing events from occurring inside the human body will prevent any harm from occurring.

Once a radioactive isotope has decays by alpha or beta, it then forms a different isotope, which is known as a decay product. Sometimes, these decay products are also radioactive, and the decay process continues until a stable isotope is formed. So the process of radioactivity decay can produce other unstable decay products.

Each radioactive isotope has its own characteristic modes of decay and characteristic energies through which these decay events occur. It is these decay modes that allow for these isotopes to be identified and measured.

The rate at which a radioactive isotope decays is referred to as the half-life. The half-life is the time needed for one half of the radioactive substance to decay into another substance. Each successive half-life again reduces the remaining amount by one half. Therefore, a radioactive isotope will decay to $1/2$, $1/4$, $1/16$, $1/32$, and so on of the original activity for each successive half-life (only for the decaying isotope—as stated, the daughter isotope can also be radioactive with a different half-life). Once a radioactive isotope has gone through six half-lives, there will only be 1.6% of the original radioactive isotope that remains. After a radioactive isotope has gone through ten half-lives, only 0.1% of the original radioactivity of that isotope remains.

3.2   UNITS OF RADIOACTIVITY

The number of decay events that occurs per second is referred to as the Becquerel (Bq), which is named after the discoverer of radioactivity Henri Becquerel. Therefore, 100 Bq implies that exactly 100 decays occur every second. Of course, the number of nuclear decays does not imply the means of decay or by what mechanism (alpha, beta, or gamma) did these decay events take place. To know this, one must understand or be familiar with the list of both stable and radioactive isotopes. This list can be found on the Radiochemistry Society website by going to www.radiochemistry.org. Each radioactive isotope has its own modes of decay and its own unique half-life, which forms the basis through which each isotope can be identified.

3.3   THE DIFFERENT TYPES OF RADIOACTIVE DECAY

Radioactive decay is not inherently harmful if this radiation does not cause ionization events or damage inside the body. The type and amount of decay that occurs determines how much damage, if any, it can do to humans and the surrounding environment. It is also possible (through high levels of radiation) to cause many types of electronics to fail.

Although all of this may seem like a lot of information to process, the types and potency of radioactive decay can be distinguished in a relatively simple way. The larger the particle and the higher the charge, the less able it is to penetrate matter. The smaller the charge, the faster it moves and the more able it is to insinuate itself between the atoms that make up other matter.

So whereas the larger, positively charged alpha decay can be stopped by a piece of paper and the singular, negatively charged beta decay can be stopped by thin metal or thicker types of plastic, such as a sheet of aluminum, it is the ionization damage that causes harm within the human body. However, it generally takes a lead or concrete wall to reduce the neutrally charged gamma rays significantly. During nuclear fission (either from a nuclear reactor or detonation of a nuclear weapon), high-energy beta and gamma radiation are discharged; hence, the concrete structures are needed to shield from the effects of radiation for these types of scenarios.

However, all of these forms of radiation are considered ionizing because when they interact with neutrally charged atoms or molecules, they remove electrons from them, which in turn causes them to become unstable and ionized. These ions also have the potential of causing secondary, tertiary, and even quaternary ions that can also induce more damage in the body, which leads to a short-term "domino effect" that lasts less than a microsecond.

In all, six types or "flavors" of nuclear "stuff" exist. Fusion products are caused when two light atomic nuclei come together to form a heavier nucleus, which releases vast amounts of energy in the process. Fission products result when a heavy unstable atom breaks into smaller parts (usually caused when struck by a neutron). Heavy and light activation products occur when the nuclei of atoms that have been hit primarily by neutrons (and rarely when hit by protons) cause the resulting "activation" product to be unstable and to emit radiation (the light activation products are formed from elements 1 to 30, whereas the heavy activation products are formed from elements 92 and above). In addition, naturally occurring products exist, which we will examine in a later section; these natural and cosmogenic products make measuring radioactivity more difficult because they occur naturally and add to all background measurements.

3.4 MEASURING RADIOACTIVITY

To determine just how much radiation has been released during the decay process, scientists rely on units of measurement determined by the international system. In the past, the curie (Ci) was the international standard for measuring the number of atoms that decay each second. Just to give you an idea of the numbers involved, one curie is the equivalent of 37 billion atoms undergoing radioactive decay in a single second (the current international standard is disintegrations per second or Bq). Nuclear counting instruments that are used to measure radioactive materials generally record in counts per minute (cpm). Because detectors are most often not 100% efficient in detecting every decay event, an efficiency factor needs to be applied to each detector. This efficiency factor allows one to "translate" counts per minute into disintegrations per minute. The simple truth is that the lower the cpm, the lower the potential for radioactive exposure to humans.

Because radiation is emitted in all directions at once and the speed at which transformation occurs is incredibly fast, most detection instruments cannot determine the exact amount of radioactivity being released. Therefore, the cpm will under-represent the true level of radioactivity, which must then be compensated for in the final equations to determine the total amount of radioactive material present (this is accomplished by using an appropriate efficiency factor). Determinations of counting efficiency are an important aspect of the nuclear measurement process. These determinations are typically done only for laboratory instruments that are not portable. Thus, most hand-held field instruments are insufficient for quantifying the amounts of activity. However, some hand-held field instruments can determine the various energies of decay (almost exclusively gamma counters) and thereby can perform a qualitative analysis—which means they perhaps can determine what isotopes are present but cannot (for the most part) determine the quantity of radioactivity present. In order to quantify the amounts of each isotope properly, one must provide samples to a qualified radiochemistry laboratory (where the nuclear counting efficiencies are known).

What makes radioactive measurements even more difficult is the concept of a half-life, which is the time it takes for a radioactive isotope to diminish to half of its original activity. However, the decay product of that material (the other radioisotopes that it decays to) can also decay and have a separate half-life. Measuring an isotope's half-life can be a vital clue in identifying what isotope is present. Another clue is the measure of the energy of decay, which is especially true for gamma rays. Most gamma emitters have a very distinct energy signature, which is much like a fingerprint.

Although some isotopes have a short half-life of seconds, minutes, hours, or days, others will have half-lives that extend past even billions of years (for example, uranium-238 has a half-life of 4.5 billion years). During the decay process, isotopes can transform into dozens of other radioactive isotopes (this is called a decay series) before finally becoming a stable form of lead (specifically lead-206 in the case of uranium-238).

Short half-life isotopes make radiation measurements more difficult if they are not compensated appropriately—especially for all of the subsequent decay products that are produced. Also, in combination or alone, decay products can have completely different characteristics—toxicity, amounts of accumulation, levels of penetration—than the parent material, so the threat they pose may be oversimplified through simple cpm measurements vis-à-vis a hand-held instrument such as a Geiger counter. Therefore, it is imperative that a complete scan include the measurement of alpha, beta, and gamma activity. In fact, it is the alpha-to-beta ratio that offers some indication of what one is dealing with. It is the latter that forms the primary basis for specific isotope identification. It should also be pointed out that instruments alone cannot be "preprogrammed" with an isotope library to identify and quantify specific radioactive isotopes. Many such instruments have been sold under the banner of "homeland" security; however, one should exercise great caution when "relying" on a machine to tell a human what isotope has been identified. Such machines (instruments) cannot predict the future and one has no way of knowing a priori what specific radioactive isotopes will indeed be present from a terrorist event. A well-seasoned and highly experienced gamma spectroscopist must be a part of the data review cycle.

3.5 ENVIRONMENTAL RADIATION

As mentioned at the beginning of this chapter, radiation is constantly occurring all around us—in fact, low levels of radioactive production even take place inside the human body. For example, bananas and milk both contain potassium, which is beneficial to life. However, most are not aware that this essential element contains potassium-40, which is radioactive. In fact, one quart of milk contains enough potassium-40 to have approximately 3000 disintegrations per minute. This does not mean milk is bad (on the contrary—"it does a body good"—potassium is essential for life), it is an inescapable fact of life and certainly nothing to fear. The nucleus is a natural part of the atom, and decay is the unraveling on the path to stabilization; so, although most people think of nuclear energy as a big concept that occurs on a large level, its origins are actually subatomic. And even though we may also think of nuclear power as a relatively modern concept, nuclear decay of natural radioactive materials has been occurring nonstop since prehistoric times.

Some radiation that exists in the environment is terrestrial (coming from the Earth itself) and primordial, with half-lives that can be traced back billions of years to the formation of our planet. Other types are cosmogenic, which are produced through natural processes that take place in the atmosphere at all times. Of course, we have no control over these forms of radiation, and we have coexisted with natural radiation since humankind was first created.

The other type of ubiquitous environmental radiation is man-made, such as byproducts of our activities and technological innovations. Think of it as white noise; although it may seem completely silent, background noises are always being generated through movement, the humming of mechanisms, and sound waves, even if we are not aware of them. On its own, a certain level of man-made radiation may be released in undetectable amounts from specific sources; together, they add up to trace amounts in the surrounding environment. The existence of natural background radiation in any form has to be factored into radiation measurements at any site where radiation is being measured.

For an example of man-made environmental radiation, we need to look no further than nuclear power plants. Large-scale malfunctions at nuclear power plants have the propensity to release radioactive isotopes into the environment. Such events are rare; two notable accidents include Three-Mile Island and Chernobyl.

However, the release of radioactivity in the day-to-day functioning of a well-regulated nuclear power plant does come close to the natural radioactivity released into atmosphere by the routine burning of coal for heat or electricity. In the early 1950s, nuclear energy was first being experimented with as a fuel source in the United States. During this time, the use of coal reached peak levels internationally. Between 1948 and 1962, eight air pollution episodes occurred in London, but the Great Smog between December 5 and 9, 1952 was the most significant. Smoke concentrations reached 56 times the "normal" level at the National Gallery, and visibility was so bad that people could not see their own feet! Within 12 hours of the beginning of the smog, some people showed respiratory problems, and hospital admissions increased dramatically. At least 4000 people above the normal mortality figures are believed to have died during the smog in the following weeks.

3.6 RADIATION FROM NUCLEAR POWER PLANTS

In addition to decreasing the possibilities of accidents dramatically, part of the reason for the strict safety standards applied to current nuclear power plants was the result of wanting to keep even trace amounts of radioactivity from entering the atmosphere. This was not always the case.

The Hanford nuclear site in the state of Washington was the first full-scale reactor in the world. It was built as part of the Manhattan Project and produced the plutonium used in Fat Man, which was the second atomic bomb dropped on Japan. During its almost 30 years of operation (from 1944 until it was decommissioned in 1972), the Hanford plant released approximately 739,000 Ci of a radioactive iodine into the surrounding area. Compare that with the Three Mile Island meltdown, which released an estimated 15 Ci of the same radioactive substance.

Since the Nuclear Regulatory Commission began in 1975 (it was formerly the Atomic Energy Committee, put in place by Eisenhower in 1954), it has introduced strict regulatory standards for all nuclear power plants that operate in the United States. Among the progress made was reinforced exteriors, improved infrastructures, a continued reliance on computerization, in-site emergency control systems, more standardized training among workers, and water-based nuclear reactors that limit the potential for core meltdowns. These advances have sharply cut down on the amount of attendant environmental radiation caused from daily operations of nuclear power plants (as well as reducing the risk of accidents). Nuclear power is now counted among the most cleanly produced sources of energy (and now is one of the cheapest given the high prices of oil today).

In addition, over the last two decades, the International Atomic Energy Agency (IAEA) spent almost $55 million helping close to 100 developing countries implement safer nuclear plant operational standards and strengthen their resources and training for radiation protection and procedures.

However, not all radioactive accidents occur at nuclear energy plants. With the increased transport of radioactive waste and the burgeoning business of creating radioisotopes for use in industry, food processing, agriculture, military usage, and medical fields, the IAEA developed several new initiatives at the end of the century to categorize sources of radioactivity and to implement appropriate measures to regulate their safety.

These commensurate steps involve government notification and authorization, as well as increased security and licensing, emergency preparedness, and safety regulations to be met during every stage of the radioactive process, from manufacturing, delivery (to reduce ruptures in casing), storage (particularly targeting potential leaks), and equipment maintenance, to disposal and the decommissioning of radioactive sites.

Currently, over 60 countries are intentionally creating and using radioactive materials for international and domestic applications. When it comes to the development of radioactive isotopes, even though safety is an issue, many would argue that the societal, physical, and financial benefits greatly outweigh the risks.

3.7   THE BENEFITS OF RADIATION ON HEALTH AND MEDICINE

Since the testing and production of nuclear weapons came to a standstill in the United States, nuclear physicists and atomic agencies have looked toward other applications of radioactive substances, and they have certainly found them. Over $420 billion of the U.S. economy can be attributed to the production of radioactive materials, which has also helped to create over four million jobs for American workers.

As unlikely as it seems for a technology originally developed as a weapon of mass destruction, many uses of radiation and nuclear power have been in the area of health, both global and individual. We have already touched on how nuclear power has become an alternative energy source that seems to be outpacing the more traditional fuel sources. One in every five homes or offices in the United States is now powered by nuclear energy; carbon emissions are reduced by millions of metric tons, which some believe could go a long way toward alleviating global warming and all the environmental and health issues caused by it.

Although nuclear energy may be one of the most depended on fuel sources in the not too distant future, the future of nuclear technology has already arrived on the medical front. Currently, radioisotopes are being used in millions of laboratories to diagnose diseases based on body fluid and tissue samples and to assess information at a more precise cellular level; over half a million cancer patients yearly receive radiation treatments as part of an inclusive recovery program. Nuclear imaging, diagnostic tests that involve gamma radiation, and "radiopharmaceuticals" (sealed and swallowed) have become indispensable in determining disease and organ function; they can embed themselves in soft tissue and often detect cancer and other illnesses in earlier stages than X-ray or traditional scanning.

Radioactive iodine has become a common method with which to treat thyroid conditions and certain forms of cancer; it replaces traditional surgery as the norm in many cases. Even George Bush, Sr., and his wife both famously drank a radioactive iodine solution to cure their Graves' disease, which is a condition that targets the thyroid gland. In addition, radioactive testing is performed on over 80% of the new drugs introduced on the market to ensure Food and Drug Administration (FDA) standards of safety and efficacy (radioactive tracers are used to show absorption and how the drug circulates through the bloodstream).

However, more cutting-edge procedures that involve radioactivity are being put into practice today. Brachytherapy is one of the most recent advances in medical technology. Sealed radioisotopes, of either high or low dosages, are implanted into the body, often into the exact site of the tumor, to destroy cancerous cells without causing damage to neighboring organs or tissue. This process can involve high-dosage seeds (which are removed immediately after the tumor is destroyed) or seeds of lower dosages (which can be kept in for weeks or perhaps put in place of where a tumor has already been removed to kill any residual cancer cells). The demand for brachytherapy has been growing steadily in the United States based on its success rate, particularly with forms of prostrate cancer.

Radiation is also being used to pinpoint accuracy in gamma-knife surgery, which eradicates or removes malignant brain tumors using gamma rays; in gamma imaging, which uses sealed radioactive seeds to transmit images of the heart, lungs, brain, and so on back to a gamma camera that produces a clearer, unattenuated image of the body; and to irradiate blood to sterilize it for use in transfusions (much like the process of irradiation used to sterilize hospital equipment).

Interestingly, the beneficial medical aspects of nuclear technology are also what make it so efficient at destroying molecular makeup—it is absorbed so easily into the body's soft tissue and, once controlled, it can kill the cells we want it to.

3.8 THE BENEFITS OF RADIATION ON AGRICULTURE

Agriculture is another area that benefits from the dual nature of radioactivity; it harnessed both the helpful and the harmful aspects. For one thing, it is used to destroy pests that can ruin crops and result in global food shortages. It is also being used to sterilize insects, which makes it impossible for them to procreate and keeps their populations down. Not only will this have a dramatic effect on food supplies, but also, perhaps more importantly, it will reduce the number of disease-transmitting insects, such as mosquitoes, which are responsible for West Nile fever and malaria (a disease that claims the lives of thousands of children in Africa each day).

Over half a million tons of food a year are already being cold sterilized or irradiated to prevent spoilage (which affects one third of the world's food production) and contamination (including microorganisms that spread salmonella and *Escherichia coli*); to increase nutritional quality, to sterilize frozen food and prepare it for packaging, or to preserve dry foods for trade and transport. The World Health Organization as well as the Food and Drug Administration are touting radiation technology as a way to provide third-world countries with more healthful and plentiful food supplies. Score one for the planet!

Radiation is also being experimented with to create new, hardier strands of crops, such as the miracle rice that helped to feed impoverished parts of Asia. Those kinds of genetically modified foods are not yet being embraced by consumers in America, where the food supply is still abundant, and the casual consumption of radioactively enhanced fare is met warily. However, producers are finding ways to implement nuclear technology into the growing and breeding process to keep supply up and costs down.

However, Americans are much more willing to swallow the usage of nuclear technology as it is applied, in a myriad ways, to industry.

3.9   THE BENEFITS OF RADIATION ON INDUSTRY

Radioactive materials have become integral in an unimaginable number of industrial applications across almost every field. Of paramount importance is its use in what has been termed "nondestructive testing." Because radiation loses energy as it passes through other forms of matter, it is an ideal tool for taking thickness and density measurements or for finding cracks and flaws below the surface.

This characteristic of radioactive substances has been put to use in gauging everything from road surface density to the thickness of the metallic coating over silverware. It is also used to find hairline fractures in jet and automobile engines, to test steel products intended for use in cars and building materials, and to gauge the density and porosity of underground pipelines and even storage containers around nuclear power plants.

On the other end of the spectrum from locating nearly imperceptible flaws is the nondestructive testing performed on enormous underwater faults. Like radar, radioactive tracers (primarily from the more penetrating beta and gamma emissions) are used to determine the topography of unseen seismic plates and to forecast possible shifting and disruptions that can manifest in devastating earthquakes and tsunamis. The same technology has been used locally for geographic contouring performed by gas, oil, and mining companies to test land qualities below the surface.

Other properties of radiation make it indispensable to industry and safety testing. For instance, detection equipment using radioactive substances is ideal for measuring amounts of corrosive substances, heat, or pressure in areas where the direct physical presence of instruments is impossible. The types of radiation that radioisotopes emit also depend on the matter with which they are interacting. Therefore, a tracer isotope will react differently to the presence of uranium than to plutonium, which allows researchers to recognize the potentially harmful substance that remains from an accidental release.

In many instances, the chemical properties of radioisotopes correspond exactly to the substances they are being used to detect, which therefore makes it easier to spot the presence of even low levels and concentrations of hazardous materials. This quality is perhaps the clearest example of "good" (controlled) radiation being put to use against "bad" (uncontrolled) sources of radiation.

Yet another quality of radioactivity that lends itself to industry is both its absorbability as well as its ability to measure other materials that have been absorbed into the same matter. Smoke detectors are a good example.

Almost all homes and businesses in the United States depend on radioactive sources to respond to smoke in the air. In a smoke detector, alpha particles are continually being emitted from americium-241. If smoke enters a chamber that contains the alpha emitter, it will block the alpha particle from getting to the detector and will signal an alarm. Similar principles are applied to monitoring the radioactivity in air by collecting air filter samples and testing them for radioactivity.

From these examples and countless others, it is easy to observe how the uses of radiation have an enormous impact on material testing, structural integrity, and public safety. Just one step away is the issue of homeland security.

3.10 THE BENEFITS OF RADIATION ON NATIONAL SECURITY

Probably the most urgent use of radioactivity today can be viewed in the area of homeland security. Nuclear and radioactive weapons were always intended to be a deterrent; now more than ever they are necessary in recognizing and eradicating the threat of terrorism.

Because of their high sensitivity, radioactive instrumentation (mostly in the form of gamma radiation) is already in place in security systems at airports, harbors, and railway stations to detect drugs and explosives being smuggled into the country in sealed containers. Gamma has the penetrating propensity; it will also react strongly in combination with other chemical compounds found in drugs and explosives.

Pertaining to the needs of first responders, the Department of Homeland Security has acquired handheld detectors that use gamma radiation for high-resolution images that can help to identify the origin and composition of dirty bombs. This device (about the size of a cell phone—which is another feature) also combines the more familiar technology of a global positioning system (GPS) with a built-in radiation sensor to locate the exact coordinates of nuclear and atomic weaponry (which, themselves emit traceable radioactive signals). The data are then read and transmitted to a network of security personnel to alert them to the findings. This radioactive advancement gives teams of first responders an edge by allowing them the chance to analyze data before actually arriving on the scene.

Gamma ray imagers have also been developed that take actual "photos" of the radiation being emitted from nuclear weaponry or hazardous waste sources. They can be used to ensure that non-nuclear proliferation treaties are being met, to check the interiors of sealed and suspect containers, or to map areas of radioactive leakage. Based on information supplied through radiation detection, a combination of sense integrate those images with others culled from traditional surveillance sources to give a more comprehensive and complete assessment of the situation.

To decrease the risks of radiological material being imported into the United States, the Department of Homeland Security expanded the finances and authority of the Nuclear Detection Office to oversee port inspection procedures and acquire more advanced radiation scanning equipment. In particular, methods are needed to detect dirty bombs or nuclear material smuggled into shipping containers destined for major seaports, with the intention of either being detonated in the port itself or delivered to an inland target. Considering that each year about 500 million shipping containers enter every major American port (located not far from major cities) from areas around the globe, friendly and otherwise, the routine trade and importation on which our country's supplies and economics rely also present a substantial threat to national security.

Customs officials or harbor security personnel require "cargo interrogation systems" that show the contents of sealed containers without making physical contact and allowing more clarity and sensitivity to chemical compounds than security X-rays afford. Most scanning equipment currently in use at domestic ports are polyvinyl toluene (PVT) devices that can detect traces of radiation but cannot distinguish between naturally occurring sources or man-made radioisotopes. This problem results in a high "false positive" rate that disrupts the commercial flow of imports and costs millions in manpower for additional inspections.

Therefore, the Nuclear Detection Office is developing a more reliable radiation scanning technology called advanced spectroscopic portal (ASP) devices, which are being tested at New York ports of entry to help improve performance and pinpoint weaknesses in software design. The short-term national security plan is to improve the existing radiation scanning equipment and use a combination of the ASP and PVT devices to reach an acceptable level of accuracy at over 20 of the largest domestic ports, many of which have also been outfitted with radiation detectors hidden inside buoys to determine the presence of illegal or potentially hazardous cargo onboard ships.

A long-term goal is for the Nuclear Detection Office to continue work on the next-generation radiation scanning devices for smuggled nuclear and radiological material. The more far-reaching objective, however, has global implications.

3.11 THE BENEFITS OF RADIOLOGICAL AND NUCLEAR MATERIAL ON INTERNATIONAL SECURITY

A few years ago, a hypothetical "threat scenario" was carried out at the Port of Los Angeles. It determined that the use of conventional explosive weapons smuggled into the port could destroy three bridges and one that connects a railway; the economic losses would reach almost $50 billion and America's ability to import essential supplies would be crippled. The food supply and healthcare access would be affected in other regions throughout the country.

More recently, however, the focus of such threat scenarios has shifted to dirty bombs or other nuclear or radiological substances that enter the country—and the resulting damage and cleanup cost could be 10-fold that of conventional weapons. To prevent these scenarios from becoming a reality, security programs have been put into place that rely as much on radiation devices as they do on international cooperation.

For example, the Customs-Trade Partnership against Terrorism, which was enacted by U.S. Customs and Border Protection, began as a response to perceived weaknesses in port security. A thorough check of millions of shipping containers (even with the use of advanced radiation devices) leaves a lot of room for error, not to mention a slowdown in the vital economic areas of trade and shipping.

Therefore, the trade partnership program takes some pressure off American port security by enlisting voluntary private enterprises among ally countries importing to the United States to bolster security measures and require radiation scanning methods at their points of loading, shipping, and manufacturing. In exchange, their shipments receive priority importing and are precleared for customs entry, which provides a definite economic advantage. Currently, about 6000 import businesses have volunteered to be a part of this program, which facilitates global trade and reduces risk to U.S. seaport security.

The U.S. Department of Energy set up a similar Secure Freight Initiative under which radiation screening devices are sent to major international ports that do not yet have them. The six foreign ports currently involved in this program use the devices to check every container leaving their country destined for U.S. shores, which facilitates import flow and safety management on our end, increases seaport security standards overseas, and decreases the amount of hazardous substances shipped abroad.

The U.S. Department of Homeland Security is testing the long-term feasibility of using this kind of program to screen all containers bound for U.S. ports from foreign countries for them to be allowed entry. In the meantime, the Container Security Initiative sets up resident U.S. Customs and Border Protection teams at participating foreign ports to determine which containers bound for the United States must undergo a thorough inspection.

Under this initiative, all shipments are registered in an electronic cargo log 24 hours before loading; this information is then sent as electronic data to an automated targeting center, which uses algorithms to identify containers deemed high-risk or those with suspect origins. The U.S. Customs and Border Protection teams, along with local security workers, ensure that these containers are screened thoroughly with radiation devices before they can be carried aboard ship. So far, this program involves 50 foreign ports, which handle about two thirds of the total number of containers shipped to the United States.

With these international initiatives in place, countries that want to increase trade with the United States are themselves primarily responsible for the safety of the shipments they export to America. The plan is that by 2012, all containers leaving from foreign ports must be subjected to imaging and radiation scanning before being loaded onto a vessel headed for a U.S. port—otherwise, they will be denied entry.

Through these programs, the use of radiation equipment is helping to constitute international standards of trade security. It is an application that, like medical, agricultural, and industrial uses of radiation, has clear global benefits—that is, when it is properly used and controlled.

CHAPTER 4

NUCLEAR COUNTERMEASURES AND NUCLEAR SECURITY

It is of vital interest to the United States to defend and fortify itself not only against the potential of an external nuclear attack and illegally imported hazardous material, but also against the possibility of nuclear and radioactive incidents and accidents that occur domestically. The International Atomic Energy Agency (IAEA) devotes itself equally to both issues but makes a distinction between nuclear safety and nuclear security. *Safety* refers to the maintenance of atomic power plants and other facilities, as well as the proper handling and disposal of radioactive products; *security* focuses on theft, unauthorized transportation and usage, as well as possible attack.

After 9/11, Cold War fears of nuclear disaster coming in the form of Russian warheads have been replaced by the terror we feel from news reports of missing uranium. And although the incidents at Three Mile Island and Chernobyl continue to symbolize nuclear safety concerns, an increased threat comes from the growing number of more mundane sources that are authorized to have radioactive substances.

With the burgeoning business of radioactive isotopes in the fields of medicine, agriculture, and industry, an increased potential for nuclear mishaps in structures outside of power plants exists now more than ever—ones that do not have the same kind of emergency systems in place that nuclear reactors do. College classrooms, hospitals, and farms are all potential sites for

Radiation Safety: Protection and Management for Homeland Security and Emergency Response. By L. A. Burchfield
Copyright © 2009 John Wiley & Sons, Inc.

calamities to occur—and are potential targets where terrorists can get their hands on radioactive material much more easily than from a highly guarded nuclear power plant equipped with surveillance cameras and radiation detectors at the doors.

In this age, the fear is less about the use of atomic energy than about atomic *access*.

4.1 SECURITY OF RADIATION SOURCES

A lack of security surrounding radioactive materials can result in their theft, loss, or abandonment—and each of these scenarios could lead to harmful amounts of public exposure to radiation, intentionally or otherwise. Each year in the United States, close to 200 cases of lost, stolen, or simply abandoned radioactive materials are brought to the attention of the Nuclear Regulatory Commission (NRC), and this number is believed to be grossly under-representative.

For one thing, unlike an intensely regulated power plant with specially trained workers, many institutions that deal with radioactive materials for commercial use have a substandard system of organization and categorization. An overworked hospital staff swamped with emergency patients could easily lose track of the amount of radioisotopes it used; if the inventory comes up short, then it seems plausible to put this down to a clerical error and not file an NRC report.

However, we must keep in mind that when José Padillia was arrested in Chicago in 2002 on a search to find radioactive materials for al-Qaeda, his targets were hospitals, universities, and research laboratories, not nuclear facilities. Although these places have less radioactive materials than a power plant, they have more than enough to create a massive public health emergency, with the added bonus of having weaker security infrastructures.

In industry, accuracy and regulation regarding radioactive substances are difficult to maintain. A problem exists with what are known as orphan sources—radioactive materials that have been lost, abandoned, or stolen from industrial sites. These orphan sources are outside of any kind of regulation yet often wind up in unexpected places within mainstream society.

For example, metal recycling centers have become extremely susceptible as unwitting receivers of radioactive materials. Orphan sources can easily find their way into scrap metal piles, because people who stumble on improperly disposed of materials (or steal them from unsecured scrap yards) may sell them for their metallic value, unaware of their radioactive content. Scrap dealers accept them, also unknowingly, and deposit them among huge amounts of inventory—much of which is sent to global markets, such as

China, who import American waste metal for building purposes. In this way, a relatively common occurrence like improperly identifying or disposing of radioactive waste could lead to dangerous incidents of radioactive exposure on an international level.

This example is more than simply a hypothetical scenario. One confirmed case of stolen radiation equipment turning up in a metal yard, where it had a serious affect on workers' health, occurred in 1996. The Nuclear Regulatory Commission's database currently stores over 2300 reports of radioactive sources having been found in such scrap metal facilities.

Breaches of radiation security have been further compounded by rising rates in illicit trafficking of radioactive substances since the 1990s. According to the World Customs Organization (WCO), customs agents had seized radioactive contraband almost 250 times within a 5-year period (1993–1998); that is 50 times a year, averaging four times a month, or almost once a week!

It is possible that these were attempts to smuggle radioactive substances out of the country for commercial purposes. However, it is also possible that if a batch had slipped across the border, it would have found its way into a terrorist cell—and that is not to say it did not happen. The 250 cases of attempted smuggling include only those that had successfully been stopped.

4.2 ATOMIC AUTHORIZATION

Currently, 103 nuclear power plants are in operation in the United States. Compare that with the 157,000 facilities authorized to use radioactive materials in accordance with the Atomic Energy Act, and it becomes clear that statistically, the larger security threat exists off the reactor sites.

Although no standardized security procedures are in place for all industries using radioactive materials, the most common form of protection comes from radiation surveillance systems at metal and scrap processing plants. Within the past 15 years, these detectors have identified over 400 types of radiation sources at scrap metal yards across the country—over half of which were discovered in the late 1990s, when more effective stopgap machinery was put in place.

Nonetheless, the International Atomic Energy Agency has been pushing for more frequent periodic exercises involving plans for first responders' reactions to the discovery of orphan sources or to unauthorized radioactive materials found in industrial environments. The U.S. Department of Energy has also issued educational material for categorizing radioactive sources and guidelines for increased radiation security on campus, hospital, or industrial grounds. These guidelines focus mainly on the importance of identifying and labeling all radioactive sources, maintaining an updated inventory, and conducting spot checks to ensure that the materials are in their proper, sealed locations and that all relevant information is accurate.

Even with appropriate security measures on site at authorized radiation facilities, this security does nothing to deter the number one source of stolen radioactive materials: the theft of vehicles used in ground transportation. When trucks loaded with radioactive substances are stolen, it once again becomes an issue of border security to make sure that none of the contraband is smuggled out of the country. However, to deter almost immediate, illegal use within the country (such as adding a radioactive element into the water supply or directly exposing a portion of the population to it), the federal government relies on aerial radiation survey devices that can locate and help in the recovery of lost or stolen radioactive substances.

4.3 SAFETY OF RADIATION SOURCES

Within the United States, facilities licensed to handle radioactive isotopes and materials must meet certain specified safety regulations. However, oversights and accidents do occur because of the unreliability or age of equipment and because of managerial or employee error. In these instances, even national safety regulations are rendered useless, although extensive first response emergency plans and containment procedures are in place to keep damage and public danger to a minimum.

Although nuclear reactors are equipped with on-site alarm systems that close off areas of radioactive leakage, off-site nuclear facilities such as hospitals and university laboratories pose a different set of safety challenges, because they do not have computerized alerts to warn of radiation exposure and often do not have well-planned response measures in place. Instead, the training and education of authorized parties often has a large part to play in the safe off-site handling of radioactive substances. However, in certain cases of accidental exposure, this strategy has proven not to be enough.

Facilities licensed to work with radioisotopes often employ workers who have minimal training in dealing with radioactive materials. Some examples of safety breaches, as unbelievable as it might sound, occurred when workers and institutions were not aware that the material they were handling was radioactive. There have been reports that in hospitals using radioactive isotopes as part of treatments, some of this hazardous material had been left out unmarked, and cleaning crews disposed of it along with the regular trash.

In one university authorized to have radioactive material as part of a study and research program, radioactive leakage was treated as any other spill and wiped up, which left trace amounts of radioactive products that spread throughout the campus. Once the true severity of the situation was discovered, innumerable students and workers had already been exposed, and subsequent cleanup costs totaled in the millions of dollars.

In yet another example of a safety breach, equipment failure was to blame during a brachytherapy procedure that involved radioisotopes. A tube came loose and the radioactive substances entered the patient's bloodstream, which killed him and subsequently exposed almost 100 staff members to potentially unsafe levels of radioactivity.

This last instance involving the patient illustrates the immediate effects of overexposure. However, in more cases than not, people who were exposed to dangerous amounts of radioactivity were unaware of it sometimes even years later when symptoms of disease manifest. (Not only does this stealth nature of radioactive substances make following safety protocol both paramount and highly problematic, but also it shows why radiation is such a prime weapon for covert terrorist operations.)

To respond to detected safety breaches, the Environmental Protection Agency and Nuclear Regulatory Commission have worked in conjunction with state and local governments, as well as with private companies, to formulate emergency procedures in cases of environmental radioactive contamination. These exercises come under the heading of Federal Radiological Emergency Response Plans, and they rely heavily on first responders knowing their personal responsibilities in an emergency situation and having access to interagency communication. Although many participating municipalities now have these contingency plans firmly in place, they do not have the means or equipment to carry them out effectively.

Nonetheless, the United States has among the highest standards of nuclear safety and one of the most stringent federal emergency systems in response to radioactive accidents. The same cannot be said for the rest of the world.

4.4 ENFORCING INTERNATIONAL STANDARDS OF SAFETY

The International Atomic Energy Agency has been at the forefront of attempting to implement global safety standards to decrease significantly the risks of radiation exposure that occur from nuclear power plants and other commercial or industrial sites. However, the agency has no legal authority—and therefore no real power—to enforce any such regulations.

Regardless, over 100 nations are currently IAEA members, which means they voluntarily pledged to abide by the agency's basic safety standards regarding nuclear energy. However, even a cursory examination of global conditions would show that these operating procedures, although endorsed by government officials often for political purposes, are not being met or maintained in practice. Recently, a rash of small- to large-scale incidents of radioactive exposure have occurred that show that these sites are not being properly managed or following established protocol.

Although no complete database exists that tracks all the radioactive accidents that have occurred around the world, close to 40 major accidents were *reported* in the two decades from 1980 to 2000, which resulted in approximately 420 cases of direct radiation overdosage. Brazil and Costa Rica are responsible for the highest immediate exposure rates—that, of course, is not counting the untold thousands of people who received high doses from the fallout of the Chernobyl nuclear reactor.

Brazil and Costa Rica, however, are both good examples of countries that may not have the economic means to ensure standards of atomic safety. In such instances, pirated or substandard building materials may have been substituted in the construction of nuclear power plants or radioisotope research facilities, and computerized alarm systems or detective devices are likely not installed on site. Furthermore, within newly developed countries (such as former Soviet states) and in the developing world, companies in the private sector working with radiation for commercial purposes do not normally have the resources to train their employees thoroughly in their daily dealings with radioactive materials.

As the IAEA concluded, even the most basic of safety standards are often not met by member governments responsible for regulating the usage and applications of radiation. The reason is most likely that they lack both the infrastructure and finances to follow the agency's safety suggestions. In fact, during the last decade, the IAEA sent advisory teams abroad to diagnose nuclear regulations that were put in practice internationally and found that half of member nations fell short of even the most minimum standards of safety.

Keep in mind, however, that this number, large as it is, only applies to *member* nations. In the more than 60 countries that do not count themselves as adherents to the IAEA, conditions may be dramatically worse.

The startling number of nations that lack nuclear safety regulations has led to an ongoing debate over global legislation. As noted, the IAEA has no enforceable authority, which led some experts and concerned members of the United Nations (U.N.) to argue for an establishment of a binding international legislative body to oversee safety procedures relevant to radioactive materials. However, opponents argue that passing a law will not change a country's existing infrastructure or resources; many nations will still fall short of safety regulations.

4.5 MEETING GLOBAL NEEDS FOR ENERGY

A current international security issue comes from the dual concerns of meeting global energy needs through nuclear power while minimizing the threat of nuclear arms production and possible safety and security breaches. The answer comes in the shape of a small, sealed, transportable, autonomous reactor known as SSTAR. This device (developed by Livermore National Laboratories) has the power of a nuclear generator but at a fraction of the size and cost.

Many developing countries, although at crisis levels for energy production, do not have the capital, space, natural resources, or trained personnel to build and maintain the most common types of nuclear reactors (the large light-water and megawatts electric structures). However, they also do not have the need for the high amounts of energy that full-sized reactors produce. SSTAR, therefore, delivers sufficient energy with automated controls, less maintenance requirements, and about 30 years' longevity before necessary refueling or replacement.

SSTAR's design provides lower cost and cleaner electricity, and it provides heat and water to parts of the developing world. It can also be applied to alternative fuel systems for automobiles powered by hydrogen here at home. The global benefits are obvious—but the crucial aspect to the United States is that the compact reactor is housed safely in a tamper-resistant container (easily transportable by ship) that does not allow access to the radioactive material inside, nor to the "secrets" of the reactor's structure and its process of nuclear fission.

Providing energy to parts of the globe is one issue in need of exploration; however, improperly disposing of nuclear and radiological waste is a problem that can have immediate effects globally.

4.6 DIFFICULTIES OF RADIOACTIVE DISPOSAL

In the United States and abroad, issues surrounding the disposal of radioactive materials impact overall nuclear safety and security. We have examined how abandoned or improperly disposed of orphan sources can lead to theft and accidental public exposure. But the expense, complex categorizations, and scarcity of disposal centers can make it difficult to discard hazardous or radioactive substances in a way that does not compromise general safety.

In America, the categorization of radioactive materials and radioisotopes used in research and industry is specific and is constantly being updated and revised—but even this level of conscientiousness causes problems when it comes to disposal. For example, when a new class of waste material is mandated, correlating disposal centers do not necessarily follow in a timely manner. This event happened with a public law passed in 1985 that identified large amounts of a sealed, low-level substance with particular radioactive properties as a unique class unto itself. This material could no longer be disposed of along with high-level radioactive material or with naturally occurring radiation products. However, the proper channels to dispose of this newly categorized material did not yet exist.

Similar problems occur when existing categories of radiation are researched, and for instance, shallow surface disposal may no longer be found suitable for certain high-level radioactive materials. In this case, a geologic repository would be required. Although this restriction is obviously created in the interest of public safety, it creates a quandary in that the Department of Energy is no longer designing or constructing such geologic repositories for the disposal of high-level radioactive materials.

Since the end of World War II, tens of thousands of sealed radioactive sources have been produced and distributed in the United States alone, particularly with the advent of radioisotopes being introduced in varying fields of medicine and industry. Needless to say, it is difficult for the Department of Energy to keep up with the demand for disposal centers created by the radiation business—especially because specific means of disposal are required for each specific class of radiation.

In the meantime, sources without a clear disposal channel are accumulating—which presents an opportunity for possible security breaches by terrorists. It also leads to concerns about safety, because leaving sealed sources to decay in storage will not work when their radioactive half-lives are long and new decay products are being produced.

As disposal sites are closing around the country, the fewer places are available to radioactive wastes properly deposit, which causes more licensed handlers to abandon materials as orphan sources. When one repository in South Carolina shut down, states on the East coast no longer had a convenient disposal site for low-level materials available to them. Furthermore, disposal sites still in operation have strident restrictions in effect. A large repository in the Yucca Mountains does not accept waste of certain classes; a waste plant in New Mexico [Waste Isolation Pilot Plant (WIPP)] cannot legally accept nondefense radiation sources.

With the threat of theft surrounding ground transportation vehicles delivering radioactive waste to disposal sites across the country, the Department of Energy has come up with an Off-Site Recovery Project intended to receive radioactive waste at the Los Alamos National Laboratory for interim storage. This project, which was appropriated $10 million of Homeland Security funds, oversees the recovery, packaging, and shipping of certain radioactive sealed sources from the public sector. Of course, transcontinental shipping is not without its own set of safety and security concerns, but for the time being, it serves as a temporary solution for the issue of disposal in the United States.

However, in countries with limited resources and land space available, one can only imagine the difficulties that proper radiation disposal presents.

4.7   A RADIATION ROLE MODEL

Since the Chernobyl nuclear reactor accident in the 1980s and the dissolution of the Soviet Union, Russia has emerged as a forerunner in the fight to ensure comprehensive nuclear safety with its 2000 proposal targeting all aspects of the radiation cycle, from production to disposal. The overall aim is to reduce the risks of radiation exposure that result from the large-scale operation of atomic energy facilities, as well as those associated with man-made and natural radioisotopes, to a socially acceptable level.

Some of the program's main objectives are as follows:

- To rectify problems with managing radioactive wastes and nuclear by-products
- To ensure radiation safety at both private and state enterprises involved in the nuclear fuel cycle
- To decontaminate and reuse land affected by high radiation levels
- To decommission nuclear power plants, reactors, and research facilities safely while continuing to develop alternative uses for atomic energy and to replace other environmentally damaging fuel sources
- To improve and update the training of radiation workers, as well as to implement a comprehensive health insurance program for them
- To systemize a consistent, state-wide process of accounting for nuclear materials and wastes
- To increase and modernize the physical safety of nuclear facilities and storage sites
- To prevent nuclear terrorism and reduce the theft, loss, and unauthorized use of nuclear material through state-wide monitoring and databases
- To reduce everyday irradiation levels at home, in the workplace, and in the environment, and to prohibit activities involving radiation that present more risk to humanity than they do benefits (also known as the "reason-ability and optimum use" principle)

Because of Russia's past production of nuclear weapons, including nuclear-powered ships and submarines, as well as its reliance on nuclear energy throughout the federation, the country is faced with a significant accumulation of radioactive waste and spent nuclear fuel. With the addition of radiation sources for commercial and industrial uses, the management of waste, the maintenance of nuclear facilities, and the implementation of safety standards have become perhaps the most important of national security concerns.

To these ends, the Russian government called for coordinated action from all federal branches, related agencies, and public or private organizations. It has also installed a statewide monitoring system that oversees the handling of radioactive materials even in commercial enterprises. The amount in rubles for such a comprehensive program comes to the equivalent of $265 million USD—which is worth the cost in safety but is a price few IAEA member nations can afford to pay.

However, for the United States in particular, the Russian program presents an example of continuing with nuclear technology on the defense and industrial fronts without compromising public safety, environmental integrity, or proper disposal facilities. In other words, the key to nuclear safety and security is not necessarily in limiting its usage, but in increasing its research and applications in ways that will be even more beneficial to society.

4.8   NUCLEAR APPLICATIONS TO INCREASE PUBLIC SAFETY AND NATIONAL SECURITY

While Russia began implementing its new nuclear safety program, the United States, under the guidance of the Department of Defense and in conjunction with the National Nuclear Security Administration, started a study (Nuclear Posture Review) of future national security needs and the country's stockpile of nuclear weapons, as well as the infrastructure needed to support it.

The study found that the existing nuclear weapons and protection capabilities would remain a key element in national defense for the foreseeable future. However, large-scale nuclear testing is no longer an option, and the safety, storage, and refurbishment of these arms are federal priorities.

Even though the manufacturing of a greater amount of nuclear weapons is not implicitly called for in the study, the maintenance and modernization of nuclear stockpiles means that the National Nuclear Security Administration's budget and responsibilities will not shrink any time soon. In fact, importance has been placed on increased efforts to advance nuclear weaponry "concepts" and to accelerate updated designs for effective storage.

The Nuclear Posture Review (NPR) outlined the main defense goals of the United States' nuclear program as deterring threats, defeating or dissuading adversaries through the use of nuclear arms, and assuring allies with our expanding nuclear technologies and capabilities. To accomplish these goals, the report established the following "New Triad" of response to national security breaches:

- Nuclear (as well as non-nuclear) strike capabilities
- Active and passive defense systems, including ballistic missiles
- Research and development in the areas of industry and defense to build and operate nuclear offensive/defensive systems

Of course, recent threats of weapons of mass destruction (WMDs) being manufactured in rogue nations make it difficult to predict, even in the short term, which future forms of deterrence will become necessary. But one certainty is that the United States must continue to adapt its Cold War nuclear defense program to more contemporary conditions of warfare.

In so doing, the NPR recommends focusing on the design of special-purpose weapons rather than on the buildup of nuclear warheads that marked the arms race and the United States' latent nuclear power. With issues of storage at the forefront of security concerns, this more streamlined approach seems like an appropriate strategy. Furthermore, the idea to convert old nuclear weapons into newer adaptations (such as earth-penetrating devices) will allow the United States to respond to current and future threats in a timely manner without having to build weaponry from scratch or to worry about issues of proper dismantling and disposal.

To ensure effectiveness without large-scale testing, nuclear arms undergo a yearly assessment based on data culled from non-nuclear experiments (as well as that taken from nuclear test databases), computer simulations, and review by laboratory design teams. However, advancement in the areas of nuclear and high-energy density physics and hydrodynamics will also help to increase understanding of the principles of nuclear science, which allows an easier process of adaptation and modernization.

Like Russia's multiyear implementation of nuclear standards, the Department of Defense's nuclear revitalization system requires a long-term outlook, which involves not only the investment of millions of dollars but also the advancement of research and development and the training, retraining, and recruitment of a top-notch nuclear workforce. (Currently, the average age of those employed in the nuclear sector is 48, which is significantly older than those working in other high-tech fields.)

Overall, the NPR's plan will continue to take effect over the next 25 years; it will result in streamlined, special-purpose nuclear weapons and in the refurbishment and surveillance of existing (although possibly diminished) stockpiles. The shift is one from deployment to design, which means that concepts for nuclear arms will be drafted but not necessarily built; existing weapons will be ready for (underground) testing, although these tests will not be regularly carried out except in cases of emergency response or safety inspection; production of and experimentation with new radiation sources (such as tritium) will take place; and new sites or pits for nuclear production will be slated, because the ones currently in operation will most likely not be sufficient to meet even short-term future requirements.

In short, the nuclear program in the United States is based on theoretical needs and potential threats that may be faced in the future. It is less a system of defense than of deterrence and response, which perfectly summarizes our current national attitude toward the very real possibility of outside attack.

4.9 CURRENT NUCLEAR AND RADIATION COUNTERMEASURES

In a recent White House address, the president's speech mirrored much of the recommendations present in the Nuclear Posture Review, particularly an increased reliance on research and development in the defense sector. He stated that in the war against terrorism, America's advanced scientific and technological foundation is what will provide us key advantages by enabling us to detect threats of bioterrorism, prevent the import and export of nuclear material, and guard against agricultural warfare. Clearly, he was not referring to our latent stockpiles of nuclear warheads.

In addition, nuclear preparedness was another main theme in the address about national defense and security. The president stressed the need for repeated exercises and drills to be performed by first response teams, as well as the need for federal, state, and local agencies to have emergency plans in place in case of biological, radiological, or nuclear attack. The result, like the Russian system of shared, statewide radiological information and inventory, would be to consolidate the efforts of various agencies and to synchronize their actions toward a single primary purpose of protecting public safety.

CHAPTER 5

NUCLEAR EVENTS AND INCIDENTS

In this climate of increased global terrorism, many individuals believe that, at minimum, a small-scale nuclear or radiological attack on U.S. soil is inevitable—more a matter of time than an issue of national defense or deterrence. Also rising along with the use and production of radioactive isotopes and orphan sources are the odds and occurrences of nuclear incidents worldwide, as well as the possibility of attacks on nuclear reactors or nuclear waste storage facilities.

As mentioned, no accurate data are available on the number of nuclear or radiological accidents that have happened—and continue to happen—across the globe. And also it is not known which form the next occurrence will take: a malfunction at a nuclear facility, like Chernobyl; a medical mishap involving radioisotopes, as in Costa Rica in 1996; a dirty bomb going off in the middle of a crowded city. . . .

What we do know, however, is that Earth will not be engulfed in a giant mushroom cloud, ending all life as we know it in a blinding instant—as we have observed in some science fiction movies. More likely, the nuclear horror will not be a result of full-on warfare, and it may not even attract much international attention at all.

Take, for instance, a disturbing news item that happened almost 20 years ago in Brazil. A man rummaging around in an abandoned medical clinic

Radiation Safety: Protection and Management for Homeland Security and Emergency Response. By L. A. Burchfield

came across a radiation therapy machine and sold it to a scrap metal dealer for its steel parts. When taking it apart, the dealer noticed a blue glow and dug out the powdery substance inside. It was radioactive cesium-137—a highly radioactive material.

Having no idea what it actually was, the dealer brought the powder home for his children to play with. His 6-year-old daughter smeared it on her face like shimmering make-up. Then, hands coated in radioactive dust, they sat down to eat dinner.

The radiation spread over several weeks, until authorities found almost 250 people in the surrounding area to be contaminated. The little girl who ingested the material was brought to the hospital for treatment—her hair was falling out, patches of skin were peeling off, and her lungs and kidneys were malfunctioning. She stayed severely sick for almost a month before she died, as did four others who were exposed to the source.

Similar incidents have occurred throughout areas that were once part of the Soviet Union. Three men in the northern Eastern European region of Georgia were ice fishing in frigid weather and came across canisters that were causing the surrounding snow to melt. Figuring they were some kind of camping equipment, the men settled down next to them to stay warm. Within a few hours, they became nauseous and their skin started to burn. It turned out that these heaters, which were loaded with highly radioactive strontium, had actually been used in the former Soviet Union as nuclear generators for electricity.

Over a dozen of these devices have turned up so far across ex-Soviet bloc countries. What is especially alarming about this situation is the International Atomic Energy Agency's (IAEA's) proclamation that the material inside these generators would make an extremely potent dirty bomb—emitting about 40 times the amount of radiation that killed the little girl in Brazil.

Even more alarming is the Russian government's confession that close to 900 of these generators had been produced and put to use throughout neighboring regions, the rest of which have not yet been accounted for.

Perhaps the most alarming aspect for the United States is the fact that Georgia and other former Soviet nations are known for their heavy trafficking of illegal items that are sold on the black market—many of which are smuggled into the Middle East.

5.1   THE SEARCH FOR NUCLEAR SUBSTANCES

Although the manufacturing of radioisotopes and the discovery of orphan sources have been proliferating in recent years, the worldwide search for nuclear substances and unsanctioned nuclear weapons has become increasingly difficult. For instance, during the writing of this book, in June 2008, the International Atomic Energy Agency sent inspectors from the United Nations into Syria to search for any evidence of secret nuclear activity, which would go against the Nuclear Non-Proliferation Treaty its government signed.

The search is based on U.S. intelligence suspecting that a Syrian structure that had been demolished by Israeli warplanes almost a year earlier was actually a close-to-completed reactor for plutonium production.

Although U.S. intelligence has not always proven accurate in the past, the IAEA is particularly interested in these allegations because of the enormity of what may be at stake: Iran has been closely linked to Syrian nuclear efforts, and another ally, North Korea, took the world stage when it detonated a nuclear bomb in 2006 for what it claimed was purposes of testing (although it more recently allowed the world to witness the destruction of one of its reactors, which had been used for plutonium weapons production). A nuclear reactor in Syria could have wide-reaching benefits for all three nations.

Syria, however, is claiming that it has only used a small reactor for the production of radioactive materials to be used in medical and agricultural research—and the fact that the government is allowing an IAEA inspection at all could be an indication that no treaty infraction occurred. But the search is being strictly limited to the area that underwent bombing, not the three other sites suspected of secret atomic activity or the areas where the radioactive dust would have settled after the explosion. And even though the IAEA agents are cleared to bring ground-penetrating radar to probe the land beneath a newly constructed building on the bombsite, it is believed that the Syrian government sanctioned a follow-up explosion to get rid of any remains from the alleged reactor and used the interim time before allowing the inspection for a massive site cleanup.

5.2 DIPLOMATIC REASONING

The case with Syria illustrates how difficult it is to deal diplomatically with the issue of global nuclear non-proliferation. As the previous chapter outlined, the United States is concentrating on maintaining and updating (though not increasing) its current nuclear stockpile for purposes of national security; thus, it seems hypocritical to launch an investigation into whether a country such as Syria is arming itself with the potential to produce nuclear weapons.

If the argument is that the United States needs nuclear warheads strictly as a deterrent or a last means of defense against atomically armed adversaries, then some perhaps might make the same assertion for Syria, who has been embroiled in conflict (ranging from a cold war to actual combat) with Israel since 1967.

So what is it that sets Syria and America apart? And why is it justified, in the eyes of most of the world, for the United States to have around 6000 known nuclear warheads and Russia to have 4200, whereas non-ex-superpowers are not permitted to level the playing field by engaging in nuclear proliferation?

Of course, one simple answer does not exist. But the differences mostly boil down to timing and intent. The former Soviet Union and the United States developed most of their nuclear weaponry during the Cold War period, before both nations signed the Nuclear Non-Proliferation Treaty in a global effort to curb the manufacturing of atomic arms and decrease the amount already in existence. Syria, however, is accused of covertly attempting to produce plutonium for weaponry well after signing the same treaty. What a difference a few decades makes.

But the difference between the late 1940s and now is more than just a matter of diplomacy. A few of today's nuclear weapons detonated together would have 500 times the power of the one dropped on Hiroshima. The amount of atomic energy released in just one technologically advanced bomb could exceed the damage done by all weapons used in every past war combined. Plutonium-based weapons—if those are, in fact, what Syria was producing—could have such power.

This advancement in technology begs another question: If the procurement of nuclear materials has become easier with the global black market and the plans of production attainable with the help of allies like North Korea, why would a nation like Syria be interested in building up its nuclear capabilities while being a signator to a voluntary nonproliferation treaty in the first place?

Again, the answer is not easy. But a recent case that involved Iran may help to shed some light on the complex diplomatic dealings taking place on the world stage. Just a month before Syria decided to open itself up to a restricted IAEA search, Iranian officials appeared before the United Nations (U.N.) Security Council to negotiate aspects regarding its own national nuclear program.

The council had argued previously that, under the Nuclear Non-Proliferation Treaty, Iran would have to forgo its work on atomic enhancement activities and stop the construction of a heavy-water nuclear reactor. In fact, the six nation-members of the council had enacted sanctions against Iran until it began to abide by these regulations.

Trade and economic sanctions have become a weapon almost as powerful as those the non-proliferation treaty attempts to curtail, so signing it surely has diplomatic benefits, as Syria may have realized. Although certainly trade between the United States and Iran is strained anyway, the import/export relationship between Iran and Germany (another member of the U.N.

Security Council) has remained mutually lucrative and beneficial to both countries' citizens since Iran has agreed to the council's advice.

Although the debate about proliferation in second- and third-world countries has centered around the issue of state rights—for example, Syria and Iran's rights, as signatories of the Nuclear Non-Proliferation Act, to develop nuclear technologies for non-weapons-related civil use—the matter may be decided by the very real consequences of economic sanctions enacted by first-world nations.

As recently as 20 years ago, there was also worldwide pressure on countries to sign and abide by the non-proliferation treaty. However, that pressure was coming from the nuclear "have-nots" against nations like the United States who had a history of nuclear weaponry and the intent to update its armaments continually along with new technological advancements. Again, however, what a difference a couple of decades can make. Now with threats of terrorism coming from rogue or third-world nations, it is the ex-super-powers who are pushing a non-proliferation agenda.

5.3 INFERRING NUCLEAR INTENT

Part of what determines whether a country is abiding by the Nuclear Non-Proliferation Treaty (and which steps or sanctions may follow) is the criteria laid out by yet another voluntary international organization: the Nuclear Suppliers Group (NSG). Composed of first-world nations that have had the means of nuclear production for a long time, the NSG decides which countries it will assist in acquiring the materials necessary for maintaining nuclear enrichment processing plants, which can be used to produce nuclear fuel for reactors as well as nuclear substances for peaceful purposes.

The Nuclear Suppliers Group first adopted the concept of criteria when officials from France, one of the group's members, proposed it in 2004. Although the criteria seem to be ever evolving (evidenced by the fact that the group did not come to a consensus when it met about Iran in May of 2008), two staples have been in effect since its inception. The first requirement is that the country potentially receiving nuclear assistance must have already signed the Nuclear Non-Proliferation Treaty. The next is that they have not breached the International Atomic Energy Agency's regulations regarding the use of nuclear technology for civil purposes—not for intended weapons activities.

According to these two scant rules, Israel, India, Pakistan, and North Korea would not be supplied with nuclear material because they have not signed the non-proliferation treaty. Iran is disqualified because it has failed to follow IAEA weapons rules. Syria's fate depends on the findings of the bomb-site search.

Of course, in this climate of global terrorism, intent—or what most nations can infer to be intent—plays a large role in determining how nuclear technology will be used and if applications of that technology should even be allowed. Rogue nations, terrorist sympathizers, governments that have advocated human rights abuses, and those ruled by unstable dictators clearly should not be assisted in achieving nuclear capability, even for civil use. However, now that nuclear "secrets" are not so secret (instructions for building atomic weapons can even be accessed on the Internet) and access to radiological material has been aided by a burgeoning black market, what steps—short of warfare—can the rest of the world use against rogue nations once nuclear proliferation can no longer be prevented?

5.4   NUCLEAR ARMS IN THE WRONG HANDS

Since the bombing of Hiroshima, the U.S. government—along with most American people—has discounted nuclear attack even as a means of defense, let alone an option for offense. Acting in good faith, the United States was one of the first nations to sign the Nuclear Non-Proliferation Treaty, and no thought has been given to the use of nuclear or radioactive weapons on our end unless very dire circumstances existed. Perhaps a large part of this because of our collective contentious rolled into our foreign policy and any collateral damage in diplomatic relations to the world as a whole. But it seems the bigger consideration is toward equanimity in dealing with nations that do not share common interests and goals.

Although speculation still surrounds Iran's nuclear capabilities, there is no doubt about the potential for biological or chemical attacks on American soil. It is also known, as witnessed through North Korea's display of nuclear testing—which many saw as a warning—that other hostile administrations have access to nuclear arms.

In a previous chapter, we have observed how Homeland Security is using the latest in radioactive devices to screen out radiological weapons or substances from entering the country. In later chapters, we will explore the intricate roles of first responders, healthcare facilities, and the military in the case of a radiological emergency. But the first crucial step toward prevention of the unthinkable starts with traditional measures: diplomacy, arms control, multilateral agreements, threat reduction tactics, and trade embargoes. In short, it is a defense founded on deepened diplomacy and financial sanctions.

According to Homeland Security documents, initial priority goes to dissuading or impeding nations and terrorist cells from achieving nuclear capability by slowing down their access to or hiking up the costs of nuclear intelligence and materials. Take, for instance, the orphan sources scattered throughout Soviet bloc countries that we discussed at the beginning of this chapter. The current U.S. administration designed the Nunn-Lugar program specifically to stop the spread of that material—and of Soviet expertise—to potential terrorists pocketed throughout the Middle East. In what is referred to as "threat reduction assistance," the United States sends economic aid and opens up trade routes with former Soviet countries willing to implement security measures designed to crack down on black market trafficking and prevent nuclear material from slipping across their borders. American allies are also taking part in the program, which was endorsed through the G-8 economic summits as the Global Partnership Against the Spread of Weapons and Materials of Mass Destruction.

Furthermore, the United States and fellow members of the Nuclear Suppliers Group stress the importance—and their support—of multilateral regimes, which includes governments that share the same nonproliferation policies that they do. Because arms control plays such an essential role in any defense strategy, the current U.S. administration has pledged to "support" (through trade, economic aid, and military alliance) regimes and emerging nation-states willing to comply with non-proliferation acts set out not only by the Nuclear Non-Proliferation Treaty but also by the Chemical Weapons Convention and the Biological Weapons Convention.

In addition to diplomatic strategy, Homeland Security is concentrating on intelligence collection about the selling and delivery of nuclear materials that do manage to find their way onto the global market. In this scenario, interdiction is critical. Effectively preventing the movement of nuclear materials through (national and international) military, intelligence, technical, and law enforcement capabilities will allow the detection and destruction of atomic weapons before they have a chance of being used or, in some cases, even assembled.

In the case of countries such as North Korea, where it is already too late for prevention because nuclear arms production has already taken place, the United States government is calling on the other 188 nations that have signed the Nuclear Non-Proliferation Treaty to keep up certain trade restrictions while maintaining diplomatic communications with the country (such as Madeleine Albright's historic trip in 2000) and continuing negotiations regarding the sending of essential supplies and technological assistance in other areas, such as sending satellites in return for disarmament.

Albright's diplomatic sojourn to North Korea occurred about 8 years ago; since then, although the country clearly has the capability, to date it has not engaged in any known nuclear aggression.

5.5 A MORE ACTIVE DEFENSE

As an active rather than as a diplomatic defense, Homeland Security is advancing its work on air and missile strategies to disable or destroy nuclear weapons en route to their intended targets. Still, nuclear advocates are claiming that to combat the new generation of nuclear arms, the United States has to step up its production of specialized nuclear weapons.

The Bush administration has been funding research into smaller sized nuclear weapons (about one third the size of "Little Boy") to be added to the U.S. arsenal and toward the further development of earth-penetrating nuclear warheads which are referred to as "bunker busters," that can infiltrate a few meters into solid rock and take out subterranean stockpiles of weapons of mass destruction (WMDs) or the underground hideouts of terrorist cells.

The argument is that, as the face of warfare changes, so, too, should our nuclear capabilities.

To uphold the Nuclear Non-Proliferation Treaty, the United States would have to modify existing nuclear warheads into more modern applications and not create entirely "new" weapons or add to the current number. However, the bigger point is that nuclear weapons, no matter how small, used to destroy other chemical or biological weapons underground will nonetheless result in severe nuclear fallout aboveground. No matter how specialized or limited they are intended to be, the result would still be catastrophic—unlike the loopholes in the Non-Proliferation Treaty, there is simply no way around that.

Finally, in the event of a nuclear attack on U.S. soil, the Federal Emergency Management Agency (FEMA), along with the Department of Homeland Security, has issued a statement focusing on three aspects of protecting one against radiation and nuclear fallout:

- Distance—The further you are from radioactive substances, the better. Generally, 95% of the United States (the areas away from probable targets) will only need to worry about nuclear fallout in the event of attack. An underground basement affords more protection than any other floors of a building, although the ground floor is not advisable; radioactive dust will collect outside, and top floors should be avoided because radioactive laden particles will collect on the rooftop.

- Shielding—The denser the materials surrounding you, the better. Take shelter in places with thick walls, concrete, bricks, or even books lining the walls.

- Time—Radioactive dust laden with fission products will have the propensity to lose their high levels of radioactivity quickly. Two weeks after a nuclear detonation, the radiation in the surrounding area will have decreased to only about 1% of its initial level. This decrease is because of the relatively short half-lives of most fission products. A few (strontium-90 and cesium-137 have decade long half-lives) will be present for decades.

To prepare for a radiological incident, FEMA and the Department of Defense have also been improving medical treatment and emergency care to focus on the particular injuries sustained by the initial blast and subsequent fallout (which will be examined in later chapters). However, should large-scale nuclear combat occur between two nuclear proliferating countries, there would be little chance of an effective immediate medical response.

In the case of Pakistan and India, both of which did not sign the non-proliferation treaty, a war between these two enemy nations involving high-powered nuclear weapons could result in over 12 million deaths and eventually wipe out the entire Asian subcontinent from the subsequent radiation fallout in the Himalayain region alone. Even a smaller scale explosion would overwhelm hospitals and supplies there and would result in widespread contamination, famine, and disease.

As of now, the exact nuclear capabilities of these two countries remains classified, but it is believed that they each have several dozen nuclear warheads and uranium production facilities working around the clock.

5.6   SHOULD DIPLOMACY FAIL

According to the Department of Defense, the most likely scenarios involving radiological fallout would occur from the use of weapons against a deployed naval force; a nuclear attack against a third-world country, either in a remote city or a nuclear production facility; a terrorist act; or an accident that involved nuclear production. Of course, with radiation being used routinely in medicine, industry, and power utilities (and the orphan sources associated with improper disposal), the risk of occupational and accidental exposure is increased.

The first reported recognition of the harmful effects of radiation came just months after the discovery of X-rays, when a scientist who worked on the project noticed his own hair falling out. By now, we have all become more acute of the potential damage that radiation can do to the human body, although many are not as familiar with the many forms radiation can take or the different injuries that different radioactive sources can inflict.

5.7   A CLOSER LOOK AT NUCLEAR WEAPONS

Compared with a conventional bomb explosion, a nuclear weapon's destructive capabilities are from the unequalled amount of energy it releases in a very small space within a very short period of time. As examined, nuclear energy results from the process of atoms converting from less stable to more stable isotopes while releasing a relatively large amount of energy—and it is this energy that acts as the destructive force behind nuclear weapons.

However, the process of stabilization can occur in two ways. When less stable larger elements (like uranium and plutonium) are split by an oncoming neutron into more stable midrange elements, it is known as fission. When lighter nuclei combine to become heavier, more stable elements, fusion has taken place. The difference is more than academic—it has been applied to nuclear weapons. The process of fusion only occurs at temperatures that are millions of degrees. Therefore, it is necessary to ignite a fusion bomb using a fission bomb. As a means of comparison, today's hydrogen bomb is a type of fusion bomb that releases enormous amounts of energy. Hydrogen bombs today can release more than a thousand times more energy that the Hiroshima bomb.

The fission component for most nuclear weapons is provided by either uranium-235 or plutonium-239. These weapons come in two basic forms: a gun-tube configuration that blows together two uranium masses, which was the design of the bomb dropped on Hiroshima; or an implosion weapon that uses a complex system of lenses to crush masses of plutonium to supercritical density, like the bombs in the Trinity tests and the one dropped on Nagasaki.

Scientifically speaking, fission weapons do not yield as much power; therefore, the megaton nuclear weapons that reside in the American and Russian arsenals are mostly fusion weapons. Weapons based on the principle of fusion combine light hydrogen isotopes into heavier elements, which produce significantly heavier damage. To illustrate the magnitude of fusion weapons, we should note that the nuclear arms amassed in India and Pakistan, which could lead to the deaths of over 10 million people and the destruction of an entire subcontinent, involve uranium production and therefore use fission. In other words, that scenario is based on the weaker of the two weapon types.

Once a weapon is detonated, it takes only about 0.6 μs for the nuclear reactions that occur inside it to release its energy. At that point, the processes of fusion and fission have already released their energy as electromagnetic radiation in the form of gamma rays, X-rays, ultraviolet light, visible light, and heat, which hits the earth as a fireball averaging a temperature of 1,000,000°. In the meantime, the products produced have transformed into a source of high energy gamma and X-ray radiation, which in turn is emitted from the bomb fireball at the speed of light. The actual materials of the bomb (the casing and interiors are immediately vaporized) expand exponentially, which causes the air to compress and results in a supersonic blast. It is these three forces that combine to cause human casualties and radiation-related injuries.

5.8 NUCLEAR BLAST FORCE

The blast of a nuclear bomb, combined with its thermal energy, is responsible for the greatest number of immediate injuries and deaths. During detonation, that blast dissipates about half of the weapon's total energy, which is a tremendous amount even in smaller-sized bombs.

The initial blast wave consists of both static and dynamic forces; as it travels away from the epicenter, the static elements form a wall of compressed air that can crush structures standing in its path. The immediate injuries it produces are the result of exposure to high pressure and winds of more than 150 miles per hour, which will usually manifest as internal bodily damage, such as broken ear drums, pulmonary rupture, and intestinal hemorrhaging.

5.9 NUCLEAR THERMAL FORCE

After detonation of a nuclear bomb, about one third of its total energy is released as thermal force. The release of this thermal energy occurs in two stages (which accounts for the unique mushroom cloud shape associated with nuclear explosions). The first is the interaction of the blast wave with the fireball, which makes up less than 1% of the total thermal output and exists as ultraviolet rays. The second, more powerful stage is the one responsible for infrared radiation burns and possible blindness caused by burning of the retina.

5.10 RADIOACTIVE FORCE

The radiation attendant to a nuclear explosion includes alpha-, beta-, gamma-, and neutron-emitting isotopes, all of which can be extremely damaging to human health in large amounts when allowed to enter the body. As the fireball begins to cool, small particles begin to coalesce into what is referred to as fallout (which are nothing more than small dust and debris particles that enclose many of the radioactive fission products from the bomb). If enough of these fallout particles are allowed to enter the body, death or radiation sickness can occur. A nuclear fallout shelter protects from the blast and subsequently from these tiny fallout particles. The major path for entering the body is through inhalation or ingestion. Therefore, if one is careful not to breath (vis-à-vis an air filter) and does not ingest (vis-à-vis maintaining clean water or food) the isotopes, one should be fine.

During the 1950s, nuclear fallout shelters were all the rage. At one point, it seemed like a fashion statement to have your own fallout shelter. These shelters provided clean food and water as well as filtered air. The idea was to be able to live in one for approximately 2 weeks (it was advised that fallout shelter inhabitants should plan to remain sheltered for at least 2 weeks, then work outside for gradually increasing amounts of time, to 4 hours a day at 3 weeks—the normal work was to sweep or wash fallout into shallow trenches to decontaminate the area). It was also advised that evacuation at 3 weeks would occur by official authorities.

Within the first minute after detonation, the initial radiation to be released consists of neutrons, which have no net charge and therefore can interact unimpeded by the electric charge of other matter (either radioactive or not and can scatter easily), and gamma rays (which, as we saw in Chapter 3, are the most penetrating and therefore can cause ionizations within a person over large distances or can also penetrate most matter).

Within the second minute, more gamma rays are released along with alpha particles (which do not penetrate the body easily but, once inhaled, are readily absorbed into internal organs and can do 10 times more internal damage than beta or gamma particles) and beta radiation (which can penetrate flesh pretty easily) as decay products of the nuclear fission process.

The residual fallout that occurs after detonation and the initial radiation is a result of the pocket of compressed air caused by the expanding bomb materials that make the blast wave. Concentrated inside this compressed compartment are extremely unstable radioactive fission or fusion fragments, which consist of the left over 80% of nuclear material that did not undergo a reaction (and still exists as uranium, plutonium, and neutron activated isotopes produced from the bomb casing and other materials), and products that became radioactive (bomb casing, debris, pieces of the ground) on contact. All of this is released as radioactive fallout.

The fallout released the first day is the most significant because it is extremely radioactive and remains geographically concentrated; it spreads out subsequently in amounts that are still very hazardous to human health. The initial fallout is made up of larger particles released within a few hundred miles of the original bombsite. As such, they exist as fission products (mostly beta- and gamma-emitting isotopes and activation products that exist as beta-, gamma-, and alpha-emitting isotopes).

Whether the nuclear weapon was fission or fusion, the nuclear event produces approximately 300 radioisotopes. Therefore, the radiological composition of nuclear fallout is exceptionally complex, and it causes a variety of injuries that result from gamma ray radiation of the entire body (internal and external), beta radiation of the skin, and internal radiation from ingested or inhaled alpha-emitting fallout particles.

In terms of widespread devastation and infrastructural damage, no scenario comes close to a mid- to full-scale nuclear attack. But in recent years, it has been replaced by bigger fears of small-scale attacks from so-called improvised nuclear devices (INDs). It is believed that such devices would be the type that a terrorist group would make and use. It is estimated that such devices would most likely be equivalent in size to the Hiroshima or Nagasaki bombs.

5.11 RADIOLOGICAL DISPERSION DEVICES

Radiological dispersion devices (RDDs) are perhaps the most controversial and highly publized type of nuclear terror device. They represent the most likely threat that America is facing today.

Also known as "dirty bombs," RDDs are considered by Homeland Security to present a far more increased risk of a terrorist attack than the use of actual nuclear weapons, in part because the ease of obtaining the necessary materials is much greater. Generally, RDDs make use of conventional explosives, such as regular bombs, but combine them with radioactive material, which, after detonation, is dispersed in dangerous amounts over a limited or concentrated area. However, ready-made versions of RDDs involve the use of common equipment, such as crop dusters and aerosol, to disperse radiation without any accompanying explosion. These types of "devices" are insidious because no explosion takes place and few places routinely monitor for increased levels of radiation. Thus, the scenario might be strategic placement of materials on food, in water, or in the air where a high population zone exists.

These radiological weapons require less technical knowledge to build or use than a nuclear bomb and can function effectively with more accessible radioactive substances, such as the kinds used in medical, industrial, and agriculture research. Whereas nuclear bombs need uranium and/or plutonium for the processes of fission to occur, dirty bombs or other forms of RDDs can be fashioned out of materials provided by the Nuclear Suppliers Group, which are cleared by the International Atomic Energy Association for a country's civil and industrial use or sold on the black markets of former Soviet countries.

However, that is not to imply that radiological materials are obtained easily, especially within the United States. Take, for example, an extremely common source of radioactivity—one that is probably present in your house right now: a smoke detector. The small amounts of radioactive elements in these devices (that attach to airborne particles) would require a huge number of smoke detectors to be amassed to have enough radioactive material to assemble a viable, high-level RDD. Before anyone could purchase even a third of the necessary number, they would most likely get a knock on their door.

We have already covered the security measures in place that make obtaining the material for an RDD into the United States via ports and border crossings extremely unlikely. However, even if that had been achieved, the radioactive source would need to be warehoused and stored for safekeeping. Transporting that material or a dirty bomb to a crowded site for detonation is no easy feat either. Even encased in shelling, the radioactive substance would perhaps cause the individuals transporting it to be exposed to a dangerous or lethal amount, which makes it difficult to deliver. Of course, it is possible that this obstacle can be overcome with enough shielding and a relay-style of transportation.

Even then, the range of lethality of RDDs is limited. Although casualties can occur from high levels of exposure near the dispersal site—and both extensive and expensive cleanup would be necessary, as well as a disruption of daily activity and productivity—the radioactive substances used in these types of weapons lose their potency within a relatively short period of time (if they were made with short-lived isotopes) and distance (given the fact that the would be dispersed—which greatly diminishes their intended effectiveness). In general, the damage inflicted on the general public by a dirty bomb is more similar to that of a conventional explosive than of a nuclear weapon. The ONLY significant difference will be the mass hysteria and fear at mention of the word "radioactive." Train cars derail and spill toxic chemicals—it is simply an artifact of living in a modern technocracy. When such events happen, people are temporarily evacuated, and the site is cleaned up. As far as actual danger and damage to life and property, it is unlikely that an RDD would be any different in terms of the needed evacuation and cleanup that occurs in most train derailments.

However, the widespread damage that RDDs do inflict is psychological fear—which makes them among the most potent weapons of choice for terrorists. Whereas a regular bomb may injure the same number of people, a radiological weapon inspires a different kind of public reaction, which is based more on deep-seated anxieties about radiation than on actual knowledge about the strength and range of its radioactivity.

Imagine the panic that would ensue if an RDD went off in a subway car, for instance. An equal number of individuals would most likely be killed in the aftermath and crushed by the tide of people trying to escape what they think is lethal levels of radiation, as by the actual RDD itself. A conventional explosive, once it has been set off, it simply does not carry the same psychological trauma.

Although a nuclear bomb would obviously have more thermal, blast, and radiological effects, the likelihood of America being under nuclear attack is remote, considering the retaliation that would ensue. And that is where the power of an RDD attack is greater than that of even a nuclear bomb—in its potential to become a reality.

CHAPTER 6

RADIOLOGICAL INCIDENTS MANAGEMENT AND PLANNING

This chapter will explain how to prepare for an attack on U.S. soil with a radiological dispersion device (RDD) or improvised nuclear device (IND). An RDD is a device that contains radioactive source material (generally not the type of material used in nuclear weapons) coupled with some means of dispersion such as from an explosive or from an aerosol sprayer. An IND is a crude nuclear weapon made from stolen nuclear warhead parts or improvised from fissile materials such as uranium or plutonium. Many government divisions have come to an intra-agency agreement focusing on the urgent need for medical countermeasures in the event that an RDD or IND is used in a terror attack. The national response to radiation exposure has been singled out as a top priority in this planning.

The Department of Health and Human Services, together with the Food and Drug Administration (FDA) and the Department of Homeland Security, has developed a project called the Public Health Emergency Medical Countermeasures Enterprise, which is a comprehensive short-, mid-, to long-term plan (with goals to be met in 2007–2008, 2009–2013, and beyond 2013, respectively) that implements the development, stockpiling, and deployment of medical countermeasures that will protect American citizens in an emergency situation.

Radiation Safety: Protection and Management for Homeland Security and Emergency Response. By L. A. Burchfield
Copyright © 2009 John Wiley & Sons, Inc.

The funding for this program will increase exponentially with each goal term and will allow more resources to be put toward the research and development, safe storage and maintenance, and use of drugs and supplies that will counteract the effects of chemical, radiological, biological, and nuclear (CRBN) warfare.

6.1 THREAT ASSESSMENT

As part of this enterprise, the federal agencies set up a system of threat assessment to establish which outside attacks pose the most likely health risks for American citizens and for national security in the near future. The top four immediate health threats were determined to be anthrax, smallpox, botulism, and radiological/nuclear materials. Therefore, for the short-term stages of this program, most of the funding and research, under what was termed Project BioShield, has focused largely on medical countermeasures in these areas. Some of these areas have already gone into effect over the last few years, such as the development and acquisition of federally licensed anthrax vaccines and therapeutics, as well as antitoxins to treat botulism.

As the public health plan continues toward its long-term goals that will extend well beyond 2013, its focus has become more widespread and allows for more research and development of medical countermeasures to the other

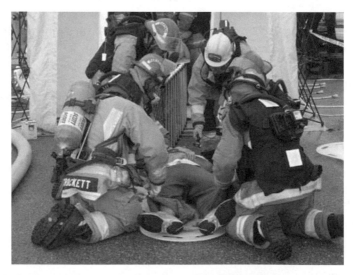

Figure 6.1. Soldiers from the 790th, 791st, and 792nd Chemical Companies that belong to the 420th Chemical Battalion and Airmen from the 141st Air Refueling Wing and 194th Regional Support Wing practice decontamination procedures.

10 determined top health risks (and enough flexibility to address even unforeseen future threats). However, for the purposes of this book, we will limit our examination to the progress that Project BioShield has made in the areas of radiological and nuclear medical countermeasures.

Since the inception of Project BioShield, both a pediatric and adult form of potassium iodide has been developed to protect individuals against the absorption of radioactive iodine. Thousands of forms of chelating agents, which help to stabilize ingested radioactive substances, have also been researched and acquired by the federal government. Among these chelating agents is one called Prussian Blue, which was developed specifically to ameliorate the effects of tissue absorption of radioactive cesium; this substance perhaps would be used in the manufacturing of "dirty bombs." However, in the U.S. medical supply, not enough prussian blue is available (which is manufactured by a German pharmaceutical company) for it to be extremely useful in mass casualty events.

To meet its medical preparedness goals, Health and Human Services is operating within the framework of treatment rather than of prevention—in other words, developing post-event responses to exposure from small-scale radiological attacks that are intended to increase the chances for short- and long-term survival. In the case of a more catastrophic (nuclear) event, prevention will ultimately come in the form of the federal government's shelter/ time/distance factors laid out in the previous chapter, and the effects on public health will depend more on national deterrent strategies than on any subsequent medical treatment.

6.2 MEDICAL STOCKPILING

The Health and Human Services agency is acutely aware that the development of countermeasure drugs is only the first step in the battle toward national preparedness in the case of a radiological event. Stockpiling enough of these supplies to cover the number of victims of an RDD or IND attack is another important component.

To that end, the agency has set up a Division of the Strategic National Stockpile (DSNS) to ensure that enough medical supplies are available, such as potassium iodine pills, for at least one million potentially affected people; that the thousands of growth factor treatments developed to counteract the symptoms of acute radiation syndrome are properly stored and can be effectively dispersed; and that a sufficient number of ChemPacks, which include antidotes for the effects of chemical nerve agents, can be readily distributed to the targeted areas across the country. In addition, massive quantities of more general medical countermeasures, such as antibiotics, first-aid

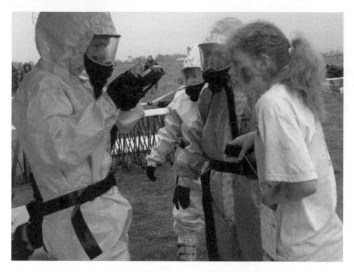

Figure 6.2. The CERF is a Chemical Biological Radiological Nuclear and high-yield Explosives (CBRNE) Enhanced Response Force Package. CERFP team members work closely with civilian agencies to respond to emergencies, search and extract victims, decontaminate them, and treat them for injuries.

supplies, and burn ointments, are being stored en masse in the event of a nuclear or radiological emergency.

Along with material threat determinations (MTDs) that assess which substances are most likely to pose a threat to American citizens in case of attack, the Department of Homeland Security has developed a population threat assessment (PTA) that estimates the number of people who might be exposed to harmful agents in the event of a CBRN attack. Based on this information, the Department of Health and Human Services uses modeling to assess which and what quantities of the available medical countermeasures can be dispersed to the public within realistic timelines (at least 6 hours).

A sufficient amount of medical treatment needed for immediate post-event use is determined based on the number of people expected to suffer high-level exposure from a single attack scenario. However, in setting goals for stockpiling, other factors must be taken into consideration, such as the advent of multiple attacks and the need for prolonged fallout care, not just rapid response.

Another factor affecting stockpiling is that following a radiological event on any scale, the national demand for treatment by citizens concerned about exposure will undoubtedly outweigh any actual need for it. To illustrate this point, consider what happened in 2006, in the days after Russian ex-KGB agent and outspoken government critic Alexander Litvinenko was poisoned in London by a radioactive polonium substance, after which he died from complications of acute radiation syndrome. When London police issued a public announcement for anyone who may have come into contact with Litvinenko to come to the hospital for radiation testing, thousands showed up, taxing the resources and capabilities of medical facilities across the city. In the end, only a handful were found to have any significant level of radiation exposure.

Therefore, after a radiological attack, it is feasible to say that thousands to hundreds of thousands of citizens will seek medical countermeasure treatments, even though only a fraction of those will actually require it. However, time and resource restraints will not allow for careful testing, so stockpiled amounts of medication must exceed the plausible number of potential victims.

Allowing for this level of pharmaceutical production will require economic and industrial resources that could exceed the medical countermeasure enterprise's long-term funding, as well as stretching the limits of regulatory safety testing. Although many drugs in the DSNS are FDA approved, others are still undergoing experimental testing, and their legal dispersal would have to fall under federal authorization for emergency usage on civilians. (The Secretary of Defense, however, is solely responsible for the research, development, and acquisition of medical countermeasures involving members of the U.S. military; the Armed Forces fall outside the auspices of the Department of Health and Human Services.)

Still another consideration when it comes to amassing medical supplies is that much of the national stockpiling of medication began in earnest shortly after 9/11, which occurred years before the Public Health Emergency Medical Countermeasures Enterprise even went into effect. That means that by the time most of the enterprise's mid-term goals have been met, many of the stored pharmaceuticals and medical supplies will have already expired. On that front, the FDA has already begun research to ensure the efficacy of the drugs after the proscribed expiration date. The intention is that costs can be kept down (and supply amount kept up) if the stockpiled medication does not have to be disposed of or even periodically renewed. Like the U.S. stockpile of nuclear arms, the intent of the medical stockpile is to maintain and update existing supplies, rather than destroy and restart from scratch.

6.3   MEDICAL DEVELOPMENT

However, as new forms of terrorism develop, particularly on the biological front, new drugs and medical developments will need to be added to the national stockpile to update the already existing supplies. In addition, more specific treatments are being prepared for particular segments of the population that are most at-risk, such as children, seniors, pregnant women, and those with special needs.

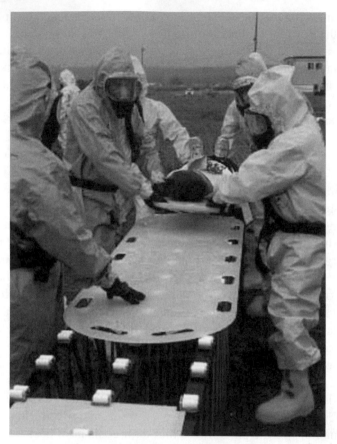

Figure 6.3. In the event of a chemical, biological, radiological, nuclear, or high-yield explosive disturbance, the CERFP team must react swiftly and efficiently. Members of the Air National Guard's 141st Civil Engineer unit are expected to respond to emergencies that occur in Washington, Idaho, Oregon, or Alaska within 6 hours. The members of this unit are part of a Search and Extract team and are the first step in the CERFP process.

In the short-term, the medical preparedness enterprise is focused on what was termed a "one bug, one drug" strategy, which means that reasonably effective countermeasures were developed to offset the effects of a wide range of resulting post-attack symptoms and syndromes. In fact, priority was given to already available medical resources that could address and mitigate what are considered to be the maximum threats of chemical, biological, radiological, and small-scale nuclear attacks.

In the long term, however, Health and Human Services is aiming to develop a broader spectrum of next-generation treatments that will target increasingly specific health concerns. A top priority has also been given to the technology and process involved in identifying—and predicting—possible new threats and radiological agents on the horizon. To do so, defense procedures in conjunction with medical research must constantly advance to keep the countermeasures on par with the actual health effects that may occur in the future, even those that, at least for now, remain unknown.

In this way, the area of medical countermeasures (like the strategy of national defense, which has to remain one step ahead of the projected next generation of radiological and nuclear weaponry) must already have one foot in the future.

6.4 READYING THE RESPONSE INFRASTRUCTURE

Although medical countermeasures may already be looking toward the future, the existing emergency response infrastructure remains firmly rooted in concerns of the present—among them, a workable and timely system of supply distribution. Even with threat assessment and stockpiling aspects worked out, federal agencies must address the issue of a viable process of dispersing medical care. For that, the Health and Human Services Department turned to the Department of Homeland Security to help improve the national emergency response capabilities following a nuclear or radiological event.

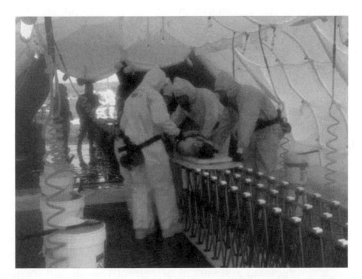

Figure 6.4. Once victims have been rescued, they are brought to a staging area where members of the 420th Chemical Battalion begin the next step in the CERFP process. A collection center, two decontamination tents, and a medical tent must be set up and operational within 90 minutes of the team's arrival. Once the decontamination process begins, the team strives to put through 175 patients per hour.

To use the medical countermeasures to their fullest, the agencies are focused on better preparing public health systems and first responders to handle a CBRN attack and prioritize those in need of immediate medical care. In addition, they are expanding laboratory research to determine possible CBRN consequences with the intentions of developing a more complete picture of the kinds of outbreaks—and containment procedures—that could follow.

As on the military response front, the medical response community is relying on improved technology to aid communication in an emergency situation. The more widespread and immediate the communication, and the more it connects federal agencies to state and local governments and response teams, the better the chances for treating or preventing radiation exposure, curtailing the spread of chemical and biological agents, and protecting food supplies from possible contamination.

In the meantime, Health and Human Services has prioritized the development of medical treatments that can be dispersed via a strategic concept of operations already supported by infrastructures now in place. In other words, for the time being, focusing on treatments that are already possible through realized short-term distribution plans takes precedence over the long term, although inevitable, goal of reworking the national emergency response infrastructure.

However, the 2013 target is to have local, state, and federal infrastructures acting uniformly and in accordance to the four main pillars of the Public Health Emergency Medical Countermeasures Enterprise: identifying and assessing likely threat; determining possible consequences and appropriate medical response; establishing and preparing medical countermeasures and processes of utilization; and developing, maintaining, and distributing necessarily supplies in the short term, mid term, and long term.

6.5   EVALUATING THE MEDICAL COUNTERMEASURE ENTERPRISE

To prioritize and develop the requisite medical countermeasures for use after a CBRN attack, Health and Human Services takes into account the top most likely threat agents as well as the risks they pose to public health; this information is considered alongside expert evaluations, U.S. intelligence, and a realistic assessment of current federal and local response capabilities.

The overall long-term goal, of course, is to provide medical countermeasures for each of the 14 top threat agents from each category (chemical, biological, radiological, and nuclear) to as much of the American population as possible in a timely manner. But in the event of a terrorist attack tomorrow, how far away are we from achieving this goal?

According to a recent federal evaluation of the Public Health Emergency Medical Countermeasures Enterprise, in some areas we are not too far from meeting the short-term objectives of the program. For instance, Project BioShield has a special reserve fund (of about $5.6 billion) available to continue financing the research and development of necessary drugs and medical treatment for the foreseeable future, in addition to those that have already been developed and acquisitioned.

However, in other areas, we are still falling far short. For example, not enough economic backing is available to build more laboratories to assess

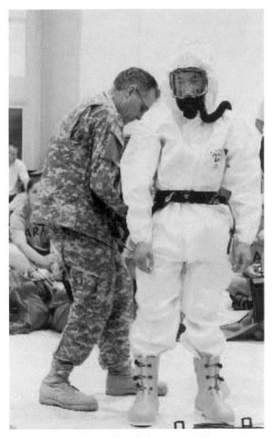

Figure 6.5. Victims of an attack or natural disaster are first taken to a collection center where they are processed and triaged. A tag around their wrist identifies the person as well as the level of care they require. A black tag indicates it is too late to treat a victim. Red alerts the team that immediate medical attention is required. An amber tag means urgent, and a green tag is used for routine injuries.

the harmful effects of certain radionuclide dosages. And although over $100 million has been earmarked to research the more general effects of acute radiation syndrome, it has been determined that no product to counter its hematopoeitic impact (which causes the destruction of blood-forming bone marrow tissue) has so far met U.S. government safety standards.

Furthermore, the declassified report found that improvements must be made to develop the national capability to respond to CBRN attack conditions and to address about 39 substantial gaps in the program, which include a lack of equipment to deter or detect certain types of radiological attacks; insufficient medical countermeasures against nontraditional agents (particularly chemical or biologically engineered); slow or incomplete means of agent testing; aging equipment and outdated methodologies to take us to the mid-term goals; a lack of countermeasures against contaminants to water/food supplies; delays in meeting future medical needs; a national emergency infrastructure that fails on physical, communicative, and intelligence aspects; and a difficulty in retaining scientists in the radiological/nuclear fields.

6.6   THE GOOD NEWS: AREAS OF IMPROVEMENT

Despite these few dozen gaps heading into the mid term, many CBRN countermeasures may be met on time with the help of other federal acts and programs. For instance, the Pandemic and All-Hazards Preparedness Act is assisting in accelerating biological and chemical countermeasures, and the Radiation Countermeasures Research Program has formed the basis for carrying out acute radiation syndrome testing on cell-based models and laboratory rats, as well as opening countermeasure testing facilities within existing institutions throughout the country, including one within the Department of Defense itself.

This increased testing will also target the delayed effects of acute radiation exposure (DEARE), which can manifest within hours to months of initial exposure and can therefore go undetected on immediate examination, which causes subsequent bodily damage and increases the number of cases of radiation exposure. The Department of Health and Human Services also foresees (by mid term) an increase in the areas of biodosimetry and radionuclide bioassay, both of which are essential for estimating received doses of radiation and thereby help in managing acute radiation syndrome as well as its delayed effects in triage and through subsequent treatment.

In addition, the Department of Health and Human Services is improving radionuclide medical countermeasures, which are considered a key component in treating health effects caused by both explosive and nonexplosive RDDs, as well as accidents that take place in nuclear power plants. An example would

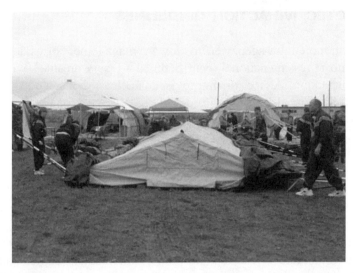

Figure 6.6. Once patients are processed and tagged, they will enter one of two decontamination tents. Those who can walk on their own enter the ambulatory tent, which is divided into two sides: one for males and one for females. Those who are too injured to walk are put on a back board and sent to the nonambulatory tent where they go through the process on rollers. Inside the tents, patients will first have their clothes removed. They are then scrubbed with pressurized warm water and decontaminators. The water used is pumped out of the tents into containers to avoid further contamination. Victims are then rinsed off and redressed in a hospital gown and sent to either the Air National Guard's medical tent for treatment or released to a civilian agency collection center to be reunited with their families. Each patient who enters the CERFP process is assisted by about 40 soldiers and airmen.

be the improved development and widespread acquisition of decorporating agents, which remove radioactive materials from the body.

The Armed Forces Radiobiology Research Institute is working on such decorporating agents that can be taken before or after exposure to radiation or biochemical terrorist attacks. The orally administered drugs aim is to bolster the body's immune system, which helps to prevent serious immediate or long-term injury caused by the inhalation or ingestion of toxic or radiological agents. The ingestion of radioactive materials can potentially weaken the immune system. These orally administered drugs would be cost effective and easily stored for use by large populations, without immediate medical supervision and would be most beneficial in lowering toxicity, resisting infection, and decreasing damage to blood-forming tissue.

We will take a more in-depth look at advancements in radiological treatments in the last chapter of this book. But as these developments above show, the national plan for emergency medical management is poised to undergo plenty of advancements as it enters the mid term. However, lessening the impacts on physical health is only part of the equation.

6.7   PROTECTIVE ACTION GUIDELINES

To establish more intra-agency efforts toward management of what it believes to be the most pressing national security threat—that is, an attack with a radiological dispersion device or improvised nuclear device—the Office of Homeland Security also issued a Proposed Protective Action Guide as a complement to the Department of Health and Human Services' medical countermeasures act. This proposal gives federal, state, and local agencies some uniform regulations to help protect the public, first emergency responders, and the surrounding environment from the effects of radiation caused by the detonation or use of an RDD or IND, as well as outlining general healthcare measures and decontamination efforts that should be taken in case of a radiological emergency.

As we have established, although radiological materials are used regularly in industry, laboratory research, hospitals, and medical centers, obtaining enough of these substances to pose a significant safety risk is a difficult undertaking because of heightened security steps. However, if enough radiological material is stolen or illegally procured, it could be used to contaminate water supplies or public buildings, which will affect health, stall productivity, require extensive site cleanup, and cause mass panic to individuals who believe they were exposed to harmful levels of radiation. For these reasons, the Department of Homeland Security has dubbed RDDs "weapons of mass disruption."

In drafting its guidelines for a radiological emergency, the federal agency looked beyond immediate medical countermeasures to a system of prioritized health-care response, aspects of detection and determent, environment decontamination, and even ways to decrease the disruption caused to national and local economies. These guides set up a methodological protocol for postevent planning and management, as well as an orderly way of determining who will receive priority medical attention.

To cover all of this, the Homeland Security protection guide drew on previously existing programs implemented by the Environmental Protection Agency (EPA) and the Nuclear Regulatory Commission (NRC) that established standard procedures for site sterilization following a radiological incident and for approximating the dosages received by individuals in the vicinity of the radiological detonation or dispersion, and by those further away.

However, the EPA decontamination guidelines on which the Proposed Protective Action Guide is based have been in use by local and state governments since the 1970s primarily as a way to respond to nuclear power plant accidents or other such unintentional releases of radiological materials. As such, they focused mainly on radioactive release in a controlled or localized environment, such as the area surrounding a nuclear reactor.

Homeland Security's renewed regulations, however, specifically address the aftermath of an RDD or IND attack, which calls for a broader spectrum emergency response approach involving immediate intra-agency action as well as recovery efforts—individual and national, medical, and economic—that continue well into the future.

To accomplish this all-encompassing approach, the department worked in conjunction with five other federal agencies (in addition to the EPA and NRC), namely the Departments of Defense, Energy, Commerce, Labor, and Health and Human Services. Their recommendations for improved response were based on threat scenarios enacted to give a general assessment of what will happen in the event of a terrorist attack on U.S. soil, such as what percent of the population will be affected, which gaps still exist in security, and how it will disrupt productivity and impact access to supplies (much of the medical information. However, it is particularly incident specific, which means the answers will vary greatly according to the kind of attack carried out and the material used). We have already observed how these threat scenarios have had a forward-reaching effect on such important areas as port security and international trade safety regulations.

However, after one such dirty bomb scenario in Seattle in 2003, each of the seven governmental departments and agencies suggested to Homeland Security that additional federal guidelines were necessary to assist state and local governments, the military, medical facilities, and first response teams in all areas of recovery after a radiological attack.

6.8 THE ROLE OF THE MILITARY IN A RADIOLOGICAL EMERGENCY

In the event that one of these threat scenarios should come true, the American Armed Forces and National Guard would be among the first organizations to respond. The Initial Response Force refers to the nearest military group (regardless of size) that reports to the emergency site, performs lifesaving rescue and medical measures, provides security and control, and reduces further exposure and environmental contamination. Being on the front lines as such, military branches undergo thorough emergency response training to potential CBRNE attacks (the additional "E" stands for "high-yield explosives") to establish roles and responsibility, as well as standard operating procedures and a federal presence.

At least 40 hours of this military emergency training is undertaken in a classroom; the rest revolves around a series of steps that together make up the Enhanced Response Force Package, which include the proper federal guidelines to follow in a national emergency.

During the third week in July 2007, 128 members of the Washington Army and Air National Guard performed annual training exercises at the Fairchild Air Force Base near Spokane, Washington. Figures 6.1 through 6.6 depict various scenarios for a mock emergency exercise. CERF-P is a Chemical Biological Radiological Nuclear and high yield Explosives (CBRNE) Enhanced Response Force Package. CERF-P members work closely with civilian agencies to respond to emergencies, search and extract victims, decontaminate them, and treat them for injuries. In the event of a chemical, biological, radiological, nuclear, or high yield explosive incident the CERF-P team must react swiftly and efficiently. Members of the Washington Air National Guard are to respond to emergencies that occur in Washington, Idaho, Oregon, or Alaska within six hours. The members of this unit are part of a Search and Extract team and are the first step in the CERF-P process.

Once victims have been rescued, they are brought to a staging area where members of the 420th Chemical Battalion begin the next step in the CERF-P process. A collection center, two decontamination tents and a medical tent, must be set up and operational within 90 minutes of the team's arrival. Once the decontamination process begins the team strives to put through 175 patients an hour.

Victims of an attack or natural disaster are first taken to a collection center where they are processed and triaged. A tag around their wrist identifies the person as well as the level of care they require. A black tag indicates it is too late to treat a victim. Red alerts the team that immediate medical attention is required. An amber tag means urgent and a green tag is for routine injuries.

Patients are processed and tracked using the Incident Response Information System (IRIS) which also uses satellites to assign and alert local hospitals and victim's families. According to military officials this system eliminates much of the confusion for both the military and civilian personnel, as well as the victim's families.

Once patients are processed and tagged, they will enter one of two decontamination tents. Those who can walk on their own enter the ambulatory tent which is divided into two sides, one for males and one for females. Those who are too injured to walk are put on a back board and sent to the non-ambulatory tent where they go through the process on rollers. Inside the tents, patients will first have their clothes removed. They are then scrubbed with pressurized warm water and decontamination agents. The contaminated water is pumped out of the tents and held in containers for processing and removal as a contamination source. Victims are then rinsed off and redressed in a hospital gown and sent to either Air National Guard's medical tent for treatment or released to a civilian agency collection center to be reunited with their families. Each patient who enters the CERF-P process is assisted by approximately 40 soldiers and airmen.

The basic purpose of the entire CERF-P process is to react to an incident with mass casualties, clean the patients and treat them so that they are of no further risk to the medical community. The hospital, the doctors and nurses, who are going to be treating casualties do not want the added burden of contamination of the hospital, hospital staff, or other patients.

The necessary response, of course, depends partly on the kind of attack carried out. In the case of a large-scale nuclear or radiological event, the Armed Forces' first priority would be to conserve fighting capability, which means that triage, immediate and tertiary medical attention, and supplies would go to members of the military first (during a declared war, all medical resources come under military jurisdiction and treatment decisions are made by brigade or battalion commanders).

However, in the more likely scenario of a smaller-scale CBRNE event, military installations, along with members of civilian agencies, are involved in determining the types of materials used in the attack, as well as locating and extracting victims, decontaminating them, and applying medical treatment.

The Initial Response Force first tests levels of radiation and identifies the radiological agent used to assess whether it is safe for civilian medical teams to be allowed in the area or if the process of locating victims can begin. Also, knowing which type of radioactive materials are present (alpha, beta, gamma) is important for later medical treatment, because hand-held low resolution nuclear detectors are generally used for on-site radiological emergencies, even though they are not as accurate as high-resolution nuclear spectrometers used in laboratories.

For high or above-average levels of radiation, a "gross decon" procedure will follow, during which members of the military are responsible for the primary care and decontamination of patients. Even in low-level RDD or IND incidents, one of the military's initial responsibilities is participating in search and extraction efforts to attempt to rescue as many victims as possible and apply immediate, although cursory, medical care. Protective clothing and masks should provide reasonable respiratory and skin protection for these procedures.

Once located, victims are taken to a temporary medical shelter where members of specialized squads (such as a Chemical Battalion) start the second step of the Enhanced Response Force process. These facilities are basic and consist of collection, decontamination, and medical tents set up (upwind of any possible fallout) within an hour of the Initial Response Force's arrival).

Victims are first brought to the collection center, which is the site of patient identification, processing, and emergency triage. The military uses a color code similar to the one used by Homeland Security in the case of terrorist activity: A green tag around a victim's wrist (which also has identification information) means that only routine care is necessary; amber represents the need for urgent, specialized medical treatment; red is an alert for immediate attention; and black indicates that a victim is dead on arrival (DOA) or beyond the help of medical science. A more technologically advanced form of communication that the military uses at this time is the incident response information system, which relies on satellites (in case of infrastructural damage) to contact local hospitals for patient intake and family notification, as well as to keep in touch with the Armed Forces Medical Radiobiology Advisory Team, located in Bethesda, Maryland. This location is staffed with physicians and technicians trained in assessing biomedical hazards of radiation exposure.

The medical processing phase comes first because often in the case of smaller scale radiological attacks, the initial life-threatening injuries are caused from an explosion or some sort of physical impact rather than from radiation exposure, so these wounds are treated as a top priority. Injuries compounded by radiation exposure or symptoms of acute radiation syndrome make triage more difficult, however, so Initial Response units working closest to the radiation site rely on unsophisticated dosimetry devices (either electronic or using radiation-sensitive material) to give an approximate estimate of radiation dosages received by victims.

When leaving the collection center, patients who have had their injuries attended to begin the decontamination phase ("decon"). The ambulatory decon tent admits victims who can walk on their own; military members assist others by strapping them to a backboard and taking them through a nonambulatory tent on a system of rollers. Patients' clothes, which were potentially exposed to radiation, are removed and destroyed, and their bodies' are checked for more evidence of injury or blast burns. Then, members of the military scrub down each individual with a mixture of soap and decontaminants, followed by a spray of pressurized warm water, which effectively removes about 95% of the surface radiation. (The water used in decon procedures gets pumped directly out of the tents into sealed containers to avoid additional cases of contamination.)

In a single-incident gross decon situation, military teams may need to treat and decontaminate more than 200 victims per hour. In the case of multiple explosions or CBRNE events, their responsibilities increase exponentially according to a more intense mass casualty response plan, even though their actions can be hindered by public panic and hysteria about radiation exposure.

After the decontamination process, victims are rinsed off and redressed in hospital gowns, then one of three things happen: They are brought to the medical tent for further treatment; they report back to the collection center where they can be cleared for release and rejoin family; or they are sent to local hospitals, where they will no longer pose a risk of exposing others to radiation.

Furthermore, because an RDD or IND explosion could result not only in bodily but environmental contamination, the initial response members must also begin the process of decontaminating the surroundings as well as picking up litter that may have been exposed to radiation.

Overall, for each victim who undergoes the Enhanced Response Force process, the work of 40 to 50 military members and National Guards is required in the form of radiological assessment; crowd control; victim rescue and intake; triage teams and immediate, prolonged, and expected medical care units; patient decon and environmental safety efforts; collection centers to identify victims and notify families; and the command base to communicate with civilian and other military agencies.

To accomplish all this, coordination is key. Effective mass casualty management in the case of a radiological emergency requires tracking and controlling the flow of both contaminated and nonexposed victims at the event site and in medical facilities; ensuring the interoperability and communication among concerned personnel and agencies; notifying the public of emergency procedures; and determining equipment effectiveness and necessary supplies.

Therefore, the military's emergency response plan relies heavily on coordination and communication with area hospitals, the Medical Radiobiology Advisory Team, and the National Institutes of Health (part of the U.S. Department of Health and Human Services), as well as the Department of Defense, local or county emergency services units, and first responders.

In the following chapters, we will examine the crucial roles that first responders and medical facilities play as well as the step-by-step procedures they follow in cases of radiological attack or emergency. Their actions clearly come together with those of the military toward the top priority of protecting public safety and national security in the event that our worst fears are realized.

CHAPTER 7

ROLE OF THE FIRST RESPONDER

First responders are the primary line of defense against radiological emergencies. Local emergency services, emergency room physicians and staff, paramedics, law enforcement officers, and fire department officers play the primary and crucial role in the early response to a radiological emergency. Within hours, national law enforcement officials will also have an important role to play in supporting the response at the local level.

This chapter provides practical guidance to the community of first responders and to those that who guide the first responders during the first hours of a radiological emergency.

The public health and safety response to radiological and chemical emergencies should be similar. In both cases, the hazardous material is below the threshold of perception, which means that human senses cannot detect hazardous levels of the toxic or radiological materials. Therefore, the initial response to a chemical spill or a radiological event follows the secondary indications of the hazards, such as follows:

- Labels, signs, or placards indicating the presence of a hazardous material
- The appearance of distinctive medical symptoms in exposed individuals
- Measurements and output from specialized detection instruments

Radiation Safety: Protection and Management for Homeland Security and Emergency Response. By L. A. Burchfield

The major goals in both crises are to protect both the public and emergency personnel, as well as to preserve the functionality of the primary care facilities, treat the injured appropriately, and monitor the exposed. Nevertheless, there are distinctions between chemical and radiological emergencies.

- Responders generally have no experience with radiation emergencies, as few have occurred.
- Very low levels of radiation that pose no significant risk can be detected rapidly with simple, commonly available instruments, unlike chemical accidents that may contain materials that elude detection.
- Radioactive materials cause radiation exposure even to people not in direct contact with them through exposure to contaminated air, dust, smoke, or liquids.
- The health effects that result from radiation exposure may not manifest at the clinical level for days, weeks, or perhaps even years.
- The public, media, and responders often have an unfounded, unrealistic, and exaggerated fear of radiation. This amplifies the health effects of the event because mass panic is a threat to public health and safety.

7.1 STRUCTURE OF THE FIRST RESPONSE TEAM'S PATTERNS OF ACTION

A basic concept in establishing an Incident Commander Support Team (ICST) for all emergencies, wherever it is located, is that the various response teams form identical organizational elements. They report to the incident commander using identical numeric and linguistic conventions so that the naming and methods of identification of unstable isotopes is standardized to reduce confusion, improve effective communication, and reduce response time. This formal structure will promote the rapid integration of response team workers from different districts with one another and will allow for the prompt import of correct resources from national resources within a shortened time.

7.2 ROLE OF THE FIRST RESPONSE TEAM

The objectives of the first response are as follows:

- Act promptly and in a reasonable manner to protect the public
- Minimize the health effects of an emergency, accident, or attack and, if possible, provide aid and comfort to control panic
- Protect emergency personnel during response operations and keep emergency facilities and hospitals operational

- Gather, protect, and marshal information for the incident commander so that the Local Command Authority can manage public health effects in response to the real problem and not to imagined threats, for law enforcement purposes and for the prevention of similar emergencies in the future
- Establish and maintain public trust in the response by including the public in the process and by opening the process to local persons in addition to the first responders
- Provide a reasonable and factual basis for an extended response in the area impacted by the release, whether accidental or deliberate

To accomplish these goals, the following three key principles govern the concept of operations:

1. Local officials are responsible for the first response as they are in the position to gather the most accurate information concerning the nature of the release of one or more unstable isotopes into the environment.
2. The incident commander (IC) will have accurate information and will be in the position to request appropriate import of useful resources from national level teams.
3. Federal officials are responsible for providing national response, supporting local response, and requesting international assistance if required.

7.3 PROTECTION OF RESPONDERS AND THE PUBLIC

Instruments normally used by emergency services to measure gamma dose rate, which include radiation pagers, do not detect hazardous levels of all forms of radioactive materials. Gamma sensors do not detect alpha and beta radiation; therefore, only a trained and properly equipped radiological assessor can fully assess radiological hazards. The radiological assessor (RA) performs the examination and then offers advice specific to the actual threat (before the RA's assessment is made, the pubic and the first responders should follow basic precautions).

7.3.1 Basic Precautions

Even without radiation detection equipment, response personnel and the public can protect themselves in the event of a radiological emergency by doing the following:

- Avoiding contact with suspected radioactive items and materials. This includes fractured canisters, broken transportation containers, and interior spaces or areas subjected to the effects of fire and explosion.

- Performing only life-saving and other critical tasks near a potentially dangerous radioactive source and quickly removing survivors from the impacted area.
- Using respiratory protection equipment within 100 yd of a fire or explosion involving a potentially dangerous radioactive source.
- Keeping the hands away from the mouth, face, and nose, and not smoking, eating, or drinking until they have washed their hands and face to avoid inadvertent ingestion of radioactive materials.
- Investigating the situation from the upwind direction.
- Decontaminating the site as soon as possible after the RA's assessment is made. Prior to the assessment, the preventive measure is dust stabilization by effective means.

Provided the first responders and their support teams take these basic precautions, emergency services personnel will face a low risk of radiation exposure while performing lifesaving and other critical actions.

On-site decontamination is desirable because it helps to prevent contamination from spreading beyond the scene of the emergency. Even if a full contamination station cannot be set up, at a minimum team members should, after exposure to the affected area, remove and bag their outer clothes; use clean warm water and soap (or a plentiful supply of disposable wet wipes) to wash or thoroughly wipe their hands, faces, and other exposed skin areas; as well as shower and wash their hair thoroughly, without abrading their skin, as soon as possible. They should also treat all materials used for cleaning (including wastewater, if possible) as hazardous waste, and must bag towels, cloths, and disposable materials and store them in a secure location, as far as practicable, to prevent or control run-off.

7.3.2 Registration of Emergency Response Personnel

It is important to keep records of individuals, especially emergency response personnel, who risk exposure to contamination. Those who may have been significantly contaminated or exposed should be tested for internal and external radioactive contamination, and if testing is not available, they should decontaminate thoroughly as a precaution.

7.4 LESSONS LEARNED FROM FIRST RESPONSE TO PAST EMERGENCIES

An analysis of previous emergency responses reveals the importance of making the arrangements for an effective first response.

Clearly allocate tasks and responsibilities. Responsibilities must be clearly assigned. In particular, it is important to assign a designated person to direct the entire response. This person is the IC. Failure to have this structure in place will contribute to an ineffective leadership for first response and will result in negative public health effects, greater adverse economic impacts, and negative conditions that precede public unrest driven by fear of loss of safety and security.

Federal officials are not the best choice to direct the first response. Federal officials are *not* local officials. The radiological IC should be a trained local official, supported as needed by federal authorities, perhaps the leading local pubic health or fire official (depending on the local custom and practice).

Unexpected or untrained volunteers can interfere with an effective first response. Because there will be volunteers and because many individuals and communities automatically move to the scene of a disaster to offer help, it is important to plan for them and to use them to improve the response, rather than to detract from it. Health professionals and volunteers have missions outside of the zone of radiological impact.

Keep the public informed. Use the media well. The media is crucial to informing the public of the factual estimates and steps to be taken in response to the emergency. There will be intense media interest; to deal with it, advise them that information will be provided on an hourly basis as the assessments are made and that the present assessments are tentative pending more complete work-up. For some members of the media, their primary interest will be in the drama inherent in the situation, and the IC has the opportunity to use the media to inform the public and nonlocal government officials about the real situation and about how to take reasonable protective steps. The media will report the steps to take regarding avoiding radiological exposure and decontamination proceedings, areas to be evacuated, and the presence of new threats as they become apparent.

A single, reliable source of all official information is crucial. This is the function of the IC. The IC should be based in a single location, through which all response organizations are given direction and from which public information is provided on a regular basis. The IC is an information manager to gather facts from the field teams, the RA, the paramedics, and the hospitals, and it is also used to ensure that the information flow is coordinated, consistent, and accurate. Without the facts, the media and the public can quickly sour. Uninformed people will purport to act as radiation experts, such as local medical practitioners or school science teachers. These persons are not trained in the risks posed by particular radioactive isotopes. When any information vacuum exists, the media will fill the void with the opinions of those most likely to broadcast wrong and misleading information.

Past failures to meet the need for trustworthy, up-to-the-moment information have contributed to economic and psychological consequences, and they have resulted in harm to the public. An informed public, however, is a trusted and valuable ally. In the past, lost or stolen dangerous radioactive items have been recovered following public announcements describing the items and associated hazards.

7.5 MANAGE THE MEDICAL RESPONSE

It is essential to have an effective, open channel of communication between local medical personnel and the officials and personnel responsible for the first response to an emergency.

Local physicians are often the first to identify a radiological emergency. A doctor may recognize symptoms of radiation exposure in a patient before the hazard becomes widely known. However, in past emergencies, some medical specialists have refused to treat potentially contaminated victims because they were not properly informed about the risks or the steps they could take to protect themselves. The medical community, which includes paramedical and emergency room teams, should learn that the risks of most radiological events have been overstated and that with simple risk management techniques, the chances of deleterious exposure to healthcare professions can be reduced to a nominal event.

Have a plan to deal with the "worried well." These people have not been injured but are concerned about their health and, in some cases, may be contaminated. In the past, such people have flooded hospitals in search of reassurance and unneeded testing. In the past, as much as 10% of the local population has asked to be monitored after the media announced a radiological emergency in a public place. The community can support monitoring, but useless monitoring from persons remote to the zone of radiological interest places inappropriate burdens on the local healthcare network.

When the former KGB Agent Alexander Litvinenko was poisoned with radioactive polonium-210 on November 1, 2006, little was known by forensic investigators. Because of the sloppy manner in which the polonium-210 was handled, traces of this rare isotope were found by investigators at several locations in London. It was not until 2 days after Litvinenko's death that health experts announced that they believe he was deliberately poisoned by polonium-210. The British government immediately set up a "hot-line" through the auspices of the Health Protection Agency (HPA) for members of the public to report if they thought they were contaminated. As of December 18, 2006 the HPA announced that 3806 people in the United Kingdom had called the direct line since the radiation scare, with 179 being followed up for further investigation. By September, 2007 the HPA had reported that more than 800 people had been offered monitoring to check for levels of polonium-210 in their bodies. Of these, 139 showed evidence of contact with polonium, and levels in 17 people were relatively elevated and warranted further monitoring. The people with elevated levels included hotel workers and a member of Mr. Litvinenko's family.

This incident underscores three important points: First, radiological sources used by terrorists may not be easily detected for some time after the incident. Second, the public announcement will cause unwarranted panic and fear. Third, a rapid and effective means of identifying those that have indeed received a substantial radiation dose is warranted. To this end, researchers at Duke University are currently working on a rapid blood test that will quickly identify those who have been exposed from those who have imagined exposure. The events in late 2006 underscore the critical need for rapid screening of the population for exposure to high levels of radiation. After all, in this case only one person received a lethal dose and a minor number of people (less than 20 showed signs of exposure), yet approximately 4000 reported that they feared exposure.

7.6 MANAGE CRIMINAL AND TERRORIST THREATS AFTER A RADIOLOGICAL EVENT

Emergencies are intended by terrorist or criminal interests to instill mass hysteria and promote fear to advance terrorist goals.

Terrorist can hide among the public. Terrorists pose a continued threat after a radiological event to emergency response personnel and the public. In the past, terrorists and criminals have identified evacuation points, staging areas, and so on as ideal locations for booby traps or secondary devices. Evacuation depots are soft targets. Rather than concentrating on the public, the evacuation plan most suited to counter the criminal threats are those with staged departures using public and private transportation over a variety of routes, like the spokes of a wheel away from the zone of radiological interest.

Items found at the scene of an attack must be treated and protected as evidence. Valuable nuclear forensic evidence has been lost or destroyed in the past because responders failed to tag and retain contaminated items while they undertook decontamination. National security and law enforcement teams will need to squeeze the facts from the site to determine the particulars of the incident. Primary materials recovered are evidence that is to be tagged to establish a chain of custody and make the exhibit, findings, and conclusions admissible evidence in federal, state, and district courts. Of value to the nuclear forensics team will be monitoring of not only radioisotopes but also stable isotopes that may have been used in the "manufacture" of the radioactive isotopes prior to use by the terrorist. Case in point, there are two paths by which the polonium-210 could have been made: One from high levels of radium-226, because polonium-210 is a daughter of radium-226. The other path would be to activate stable bismuth-209 in a nuclear reactor to make bismuth-210 (the precursor of polonium-210). Analyzing for both stable and radioactive isotopes may perhaps help investigators determine the path and thereby the level of sophistication needed in preparation of the radiological terror device.

7.7 LAUNCHING THE FIRST RESPONSE

The first response is usually triggered by a report of a potential radiological emergency, or when a terrorist group or individual threatens an attack using radioactive material. This information is typically received by a local emergency dispatch center called the response initiator. This is a 24/7 operation, such as the 911-emergency dispatcher who serves the local police station or fire department. Often the warning will also be provided to the media. The media should be advised to provide the threat information to the response initiator forthwith.

It is the response initiator who gets basic information about the emergency, provides initial advice to the caller, calls on the national emergency operations center (EOC) for help in assessing the threat, and immediately dispatches local emergency services personnel to the scene of the potential emergency.

Emergency first responders include law enforcement, fire department, and emergency medical services (EMS). It is unlikely that these responders will have either the experience or the equipment to assess radiological hazards. Therefore, they must assume that a radiological hazard exists until it is assessed and confirmed or rejected by a radiological assessor, and they must take steps to protect themselves and the public.

7.8 INCIDENT COMMAND

As soon as the initial emergency response team arrives at the site of the emergency, the senior member of the department supporting the field team becomes the de facto initial IC. In the case of a radiological emergency, this would be the fire department chief or lead local law enforcement officer.

To ensure a coordinated response, the incident command system (ICS) must have a single IC, supported by a command group. However, if the emergency involves several jurisdictions or has national implications, the position of IC may pass to a qualified local or national official, possibly supported by a command group comprising representatives of local and national organizations.

The IC's first responsibility is to set up the incident command post (ICP) at a safe and secure location near and upwind of the emergency scene. Once the ICP is set up, the IC must evaluate and begin to coordinate the response to the emergency:

- Direct local resources as needed.
- Invoke the national EOC for national support, such as a radiological assessor, which should arrive within a day. National officials should base themselves at the ICP and coordinate with local officials to address national issues. The local RA should be in charge of the sample gathering team at the site to make the preliminary assessment as to the identity, quantity, and nature of the isotopes present in the environment.
- Take steps to protect emergency response personnel, the public, and evidence in the case of terrorist or criminal activity. The review of the basics should be undertaken on the way to the field.
- Appoint a local public information officer (PIO) to coordinate local and national officials with the media and keep the public informed to support the information flow from the IC to the media at hourly briefings (which will also advise members of the public of the basics and what to do to protect their own safety).
- Local hospitals and clinics are warned of the probable influx of people needing treatment so that they can set up cordons and entry controls and can make arrangements to care for the injured or those exposed.
- The media typically begins live reporting nationally and locally within hours of the start of the emergency, so the PIO must ensure that they receive useful, understandable, and consistent information from a single local source. There must be unity in the message and a frank assessment of the facts as determined by the RA.

7.9 MEMBERS OF THE FIRST RESPONSE TEAM

All emergency response activities demand coordinated planning. The IC establishes a team to plan, obtain, and coordinate the resources.

The resource coordinator (RC) is responsible for establishing the staging area, determining what resources are necessary, and putting out the call for the basics, which include showers from hydrants, soap, and change of clothing; requesting needed assistance; integrating that assistance with the volunteers and resources that were not requested (the "extras" can participate by providing services in support of the relief effort, such as transportation or surveillance); and providing cell phone conference node numbers to the team members and the "para-extras."

A 24-hour planning coordinator is responsible for developing incident action plans, which define response activities and allocate resources for the first 12 to 24 hours, as well as the remainder of the emergency phase and long-term recovery. An operations function implements response activities in accordance with these plans.

For a small emergency, the IC may direct operations. In a complex response, or for events with several areas of operations, the IC may appoint on-scene controllers to provide more localized response management. They are responsible for the operational management of response actions at the scene of an emergency. They report to the IC and are usually the senior member of the on-scene response teams.

The fire department is typically responsible for establishing the innercordoned area; performing search and rescue operations; triage and first aid (until relieved by the EMS); dealing with conventional hazards (e.g., fires and hazardous materials); responder accountability; and processing, registration, monitoring, and decontamination of the public and responders.

The EMS is responsible for providing on-site medical response, advising medical transport and local receiving hospitals on the risks and appropriate protective actions to take, and establishing a temporary morgue.

A law-enforcement/security team is typically responsible for establishing the security perimeter; providing security for areas outside the security perimeter, including the ICP, hospital, staging area and public information center (PIC); providing security at public registration, triage/first aid, and monitoring and decontamination areas; and managing evidence until relieved by the nuclear forensics evidence management team (nFEMT).

The nFEMT is responsible for: gathering, examining, and controlling evidence; disseminating information and intelligence recovered from the scene through the IC; setting priorities and formulating a strategy to investigate the scene.

A first responder responsible for radiological monitoring may be sourced from a local user of radioactive material (e.g., hospital, university, and research reactor). They may not be qualified as a radiological assessors but can use basic radiation monitoring instruments to perform simple assessment tasks. They must be equipped with available detectors and the lines of communication to the trained and professional RAs.

A radiological assessor or team will usually not be available for at least several hours. These persons will be in contact with the first responders during the first moments of the situation. They are trained, equipped, and qualified to assess alpha-, beta-, neutron-, and gamma-emitting material; perform radiation surveys and dose assessments; control contamination; ensure radiation protection of emergency workers; recommend protective actions; and provide radiation protection support.

Other functions, such as logistics, finance, and administration, may also be needed.

A weakness that most scenarios have not addressed is the planning for sample management and logistical support for specialized radiochemistry analysis. Many state and even federal laboratories are not equipped with the specialized equipment that will be utilized for measuring radiological samples. Also, those radiochemistry laboratories that are generally not prepared for analyzing the hundreds of samples that may be important to a large radiological event. As a result, staging, logistics, and coordination of all radiological samples being flown to numerous laboratories will be a significant challenge that has not been adequately addressed with most staged or mock radiological events.

7.10 PRELIMINARY ASSESSMENT AND RESPONSE

On arrival at the scene of a radiological emergency, first responders should first assess the situation and radiological hazard. Based on this assessment, they should cordon off the area. A safety perimeter cordons off the dangerous radioactive source and indicates that precautions are needed to protect responders and the public from exposure and contamination. A security perimeter beyond the safety perimeter is also set up as the boundary of the area that is controlled for security reasons, especially in the case of criminal or terrorist activity.

The size of the safety area is based initially on visual information, such as markings caused by an explosion. As data on ambient radiation readings become available, this area may be revised. It is important to err on the side of caution; only a radiological assessor can assess the entire radiological hazard and reduce the boundaries of the inner cordoned area. Prevailing winds near the event can define the boundaries of the maximum area of radioactive interest. Additionally, it is important to note that some types of radioactive materials can escape detection, which is especially true of alpha-emitting radionuclides. As a result, guidelines for security barriers are a basis for expansion only of the safety zone and are not intended for reduction of the safety zone.

The actual boundaries of the initial safety and security perimeters should be easily recognizable and secured, and the safety perimeter should be established at least as far from the source as indicated in Table 7.1, until the radiological assessor has assessed the situation with field data.

TABLE 7.1. Recommended Radius of Safety Zone for Radiological Emergency

Condition	Safety Area Radius
Initial Outdoor Conditions	
Unshielded or potentially damaged radioactive source	100 ft or 30 m
Suspected liquid radiological source	110 yd or 100 m
Burned area involving fumes from suspected radioactive source	330 yd or 300 m
Exploded bomb or unexploded device suspected of being a radiological dispersion device	0.25 mi or 400 m
Initial Indoor Conditions	
Damage or spill of potential radiological source	Evacuate affected floor and floors above or below affected area
Fire or explosion of suspected radiological device	Evacuation of entire building
Expanded Radiological Monitoring	
100 μSv/hr at 3 ft above ground level	Expand radius as necessary until below 100 μSv/hr

7.11 EMERGENCY RESPONSE TEAM

The entire emergency response team falls under the IC's leadership with regard to any work relating to the emergency. This includes community services, such as police, fire department, hospitals, ambulance services, and national response teams.

Everyone involved in the emergency response is responsible, to at least some extent, for executing the following actions: (1) following the personnel protection guidelines to protect their own safety, as well as remembering and advising fellow responders that the risk from a contaminated person is negligible if they follow these guidelines; (2) consistently giving serious medical problems priority over radiological concerns and recognizing that those who can respond to a voice announcement to come to the gathering point can probably wait for medical attention; (3) being regularly monitored if exposed to contamination, and if contaminated to levels more than 0.3 μSv/hr, getting decontaminated promptly by showering and changing clothes; (4) when relieved of their duties in a contaminated area, not leaving the perimeter until being decontaminated at the response center contamination control area; and (5) keeping good records of emergency workers entering the secure area, evacuees, the injured, the decontaminated, and those who test positive for contamination.

When dealing with contaminated clothing and personal items, emergency response teams are responsible for double-bagging clothing and putting personal items in a sealed plastic bag; issuing a receipt for anything they do not return to the owner; as well as storing bagged contaminated items in an isolated and secure location, such as a locking dumpster.

Furthermore, it is their role to do the following: (1) treat the scene as a crime scene until it is proven otherwise and treat records, such as monitoring results and registration forms, as well as contaminated items, as evidence; (2) coordinate their activities with the law enforcement or security teams and nFEMT; (3) respond as indicated to the RA; (4) provide people with information on where to get more instructions after they are released, and advise them to listen for and follow official instructions provided through the media; (5) help to prevent panic and ensure an effective emergency response by making sure that people understand the extent of the risk they are exposed to and that, even if contaminated, they can take action to protect themselves; (6) advise the "worried well" not to go to the hospital, but to use the facility set up for their monitoring and reassurance by the IC away from local hospitals and physicians' offices; (7) keep the PIO informed about developments relating to the emergency response and direct media inquires to the PIO; (8) assess their team's needs and request additional resources if needed; and (9) ensure that volunteers and others are searched for weapons before being decontaminated if terrorism or criminal activity is suspected, to protect emergency workers from potentially armed suspects.

People responsible for monitoring radioactive areas and equipment must be aware that some instruments can be saturated by very high radiation levels. As a result, they show a low or zero reading in dangerous areas. To ensure accurate readings, they should approach the scene with an instrument that can read at least $100\,\mathrm{mSv/hr}$, switch on the instrument before approaching to begin reading at below saturation level, and avoid areas with ambient dose rates greater than $100\,\mathrm{mSv/hr}$.

7.12 INCIDENT COMMANDER ACTION GUIDE

In the event of potential or actual significant public external exposure to radioactive contamination, the senior first responder assumes the role of IC until relieved. Their responsibilities are as follows: (1) protect the team; (2) observe, assess, and respond to the situation; (3) save lives and prevent escalation; (4) extend the response, as needed; and (5) record all their decisions.

7.12.1 Observe and Assess

The IC should observe the site of the incident from a distance of at least 30 yd and look for the following:

- Possible radiological and other hazards
- People at risk
- Security concerns, such as armed individuals and explosives
- Signs, placards, labels, markings, or United Nations numbers that indicate dangerous or radioactive materials may be in the vicinity

To assess the situation, the IC should define the cordoned safety area and should reposition personnel, vehicles, and equipment accordingly. (Indications of a possible radiological hazard and of a dangerous source are described in the next section—*Action Plan.*)

In the case of criminal or terrorist activity, the IC must assume that the perpetrators are among the public and must avoid using mobile phones and radio communications until the area has been cleared of explosives, secondary devices, and booby traps.

7.12.2 Save Lives and Prevent Escalation

The IC must implement rescue activities with the priority of rescuing people in life-threatening situations, regardless of the presence of radioactive contamination.

To do this, it is necessary to do the following: (1) establish and mark the safety perimeter, limit entry to response personnel only, and keep account of personnel; (2) establish an ICP and a staging area outside the inner perimeter; (3) evacuate the public as quickly as possible, assuming that people from the area are contaminated; (4) conduct interviews to locate suspected radioactive devices and to identify possibly exposed individuals; (5) deal with serious conventional hazards (e.g., fire); (6) implement whatever steps are necessary and practicable to control contamination; (7) treat the scene as a crime scene, until it is proven otherwise; (8) coordinate activities with the law enforcement and security teams and nFEMT; (9) make public announcements to reduce the number of "worried well" going to the local hospital; and (10) advise the public to limit their use of public transport that may be contaminated, until it has been evaluated by the RA.

7.12.3 Extend the Response

Periodically, during the course of emergency operations, the IC should re-evaluate the initial response, including the following:

- Having the RC assess and obtain needed resources, as well as develop a 24-hour plan.

- Ensuring that individuals with specific responsibilities are fulfilling their functions.
- Confirming that responders are following the personnel protection guidelines and that the public protection guidelines have been implemented.
- Considering the possibility of a second event. It is not advisable to commit all resources entirely to one event. The response should be staged assuming that more events are in the offing.
- Not attempting evidence recovery or decontamination of the scene until the recovery plan is prepared and the RA has implemented procedures to control the dose.
- Coordinating with the nFEMT, if applicable.
- For a major emergency, forming a command group and preparing for long-term operations.

7.13 RESOURCE COORDINATOR ACTION GUIDE

The RC's primary role is to support the IC and to coordinate all the resources available for dealing with the emergency, which include resources that have not been specifically requested, such as volunteers from the community. To fulfill this function, it is essential to set up a secure staging area. From this base, the RC will do the following: (1) integrate all resources into the rescue process; determine what resources and personnel are needed, confirm these with the IC, and obtain the resources; (2) ensure that all responders understand the organization and know how to follow the personnel protection guidelines; (3) establish means to communicate with responders on the scene to get information on additional resources needed; and (4) collect and retain records of the responders and members of the public.

Where mass casualties occur, the RC supports EMS and requests aid from other agencies, which include transportation sources. Working with relevant organizations, the RC also helps to establish a secure secondary location for monitoring and reassuring the "worried well." Periodically, the RC, in coordination with the IC, reviews the resources from the perspective of a 24-hour planned operation and requests assistance as needed.

7.14 FIRE DEPARTMENTS ACTION GUIDE

Members of the fire department should wear standard fire fighting protective clothing and select the highest level of respiratory protection available. Apart from fire control, they are also responsible for helping to establish the safety perimeter. Using standard search and rescue and fire-fighting operating procedures, they should account for personnel within the inner cordoned area, perform contamination control for those entering or leaving the inner cordoned area, and evacuate the people from the inner cordoned area.

While dealing with conventional hazards, they must also provide first aid and triage until relieved by EMS, and they must register, monitor, and decontaminate people evacuated from the inner cordoned area using water tapped from fire hydrants for the first field decontamination after fire, if any is controlled.

If the situation requires security—for instance, in the case of criminal or terrorist activity—the fire department is responsible for coordinating with law enforcement. The security perimeter is established with the police teams controlling the outside of the perimeter line and the fire and emergency medical teams both under the control of the IC in the inner perimeter.

7.15 EMERGENCY MEDICAL SERVICE ACTION GUIDE

The EMS is responsible for following standard operating procedures as far as possible to implement and manage the on-scene medical response. They are briefed by the IC or by the lead medical professional.

EMS workers must not delay lifesaving actions because of the presence of radioactive materials or delay the transport of seriously injured victims because of decontamination procedures. To control the spread of contamination, EMS workers should remove victims' outer clothing, wrap the victims in blankets, and tag the victims as possibly contaminated using colored tape or other suitable markers.

They are also responsible for the following: (1) first aid and field triage, and managing the first aid/triage area; (2) working with hospitals to arrange for transport and treatment of all injuries requiring hospitalization, giving priority to life-threatening injuries; and (3) setting up a temporary secured morgue away from public view.

The "worried well" need to be sent to a separate location, where uninjured people who are concerned about radiation can be monitored and reassured. Setting up this location is the responsibility of the RC, but EMTs may have to bring the need for it to the RC's attention.

In dealing with receiving hospitals, medical transport, and other caregiver personnel, EMTs should know the following: (1) how to protect themselves and limit the spread of contamination; (2) that the risk from a contaminated patient is negligible, if they take the necessary basic steps to avoid contamination; and (3) that efforts to limit the spread of contamination should not interfere with lifesaving actions.

7.16   LAW ENFORCEMENT/SECURITY TEAM ACTION GUIDE

The law enforcement and security teams follow standard operating procedures as far as possible to maintain security and protect evidence during a radiological emergency. Their primary responsibility is to establish and maintain a security perimeter, which cordons off an area beyond the safety perimeter defined by the IC. In addition, they secure the response facilities, including the ICP, staging area, and PIC, which are located outside the safety perimeter.

In performing their duties, law enforcement and security personnel must treat the scene as a crime scene until it is proven otherwise, cooperate with other response personnel, and not interfere with lifesaving operations.

For a security event, they must check for suspects, terrorists, booby traps, and other potentially harmful devices, as well as protecting responders interacting with the public within public registration, triage/first aid, monitoring, and decontamination areas both at receiving hospitals and during medical transport.

Their roles are also to do the following: (1) maintain open transportation corridors to the hospital(s); (2) search evacuees for weapons before registration, monitoring, decontamination, and transport, without interfering with lifesaving actions by other response personnel; (3) preserve evidence and identify or apprehend possible suspects; (4) prevent/suppress possible criminal acts at the scene, such as theft or destruction of documents or evidence; (5) in cooperation with local hospitals and EMS, cordon the area around local hospitals to redirect uninjured individuals who come to the hospital to the "away" location established by the RC, for monitoring and reassuring the "worried well"; and (6) gather security information for the IC.

7.17   FORENSIC EVIDENCE MANAGEMENT TEAM ACTION GUIDE

The primary responsibility of the nFEMT is to develop and formulate the strategy to examine the scene and recover evidence. It must follow normal crime scene procedures, which are adjusted to treat all materials as potentially contaminated or radioactive until they have been assessed by the RA.

The nFEMT coordinates with other response teams without interfering with lifesaving operations. It includes representatives from major response teams and functions, including medical, law enforcement, and first responder monitor or a member from the radiological assessment team. Working with the RA, they establish a secure forensic evidence management area and, from this location, manage the recovery, protection, and removal of evidence. This involves the following:

- Instructing other response teams to preserve evidence (monitoring results, clothing, etc.), without compromising safety
- Collecting, handling, and labeling evidence safely
- Photographing and recording evidence *in situ* before removal
- Packing evidence for future forensic examination

Working with receiving hospitals, the nFEMT establishes protocols for examining injured people to identify and recover evidence from the scene. This includes making arrangements for blood samples to be taken before transfusion; X-ray examination; recovery of evidence, such as foreign objects removed during surgery; and recovery of monitoring results or contaminated clothing.

It must also establish protocols with the local hospitals or morgue for examination of human remains to identify and recover any evidence from the scene. This includes making arrangements for retaining the bodies until they have been examined for forensic evidence; X-ray examination; and a nFEMT member to be present during any post mortem examination, to collect evidence and maintain the chain of custody.

7.18   PUBLIC INFORMATION OFFICER ACTION GUIDE

The PIO's primary responsibility is to provide the public with useful, timely, truthful, consistent, and appropriate information throughout an emergency. The PIO works with the law enforcement team to prepare for immense media attention, which includes the arrival of reporters at the scene. The PIO is the official source of public information, and the IC informs the on-scene responders, law enforcement officials, hospitals, local government, and national EOC to refer media inquires to the PIO.

In addition, the PIO works with the IC to develop and issue a press release, which describes the event and the threat of follow-ups and the ideal that the radiation contamination is local and will not move. Also, the press release will describe appropriate and inappropriate public response actions and actions being taken to ensure public safety and protection of property.

As soon as possible, the PIO establishes a PIC, where they hold media briefings. Qualified spokespersons, or panels with representatives of all organizations involved in the response, should provide the briefings. Representatives of local and national governments should be included in these briefings. The PIO must also prepare for international inquiries and provide rumor control.

7.19 CRISIS COMMUNICATION TIPS

In their role as spokesperson, the PIO must stay within their scope of responsibilities, tell the truth and be transparent, and ensure that a single official message is delivered. To achieve this, it is important to do the following: (1) avoid using technical terms and attempts to over-reassure; (2) acknowledge uncertainty; (3) where information is not available, express a wish to provide answers, and explain the process in place to find answers; (4) acknowledge people's fears; (5) and give people things to do.

The PIO must be prepared to answer questions such as following:

- Are my family and I safe?
- What can I do to protect my family and myself?
- Who is in charge?
- What happened?
- How did this happen?
- What else can go wrong?

While dealing with questions, however, the PIO must stay on message, in part by repeating important points. Useful phrases include the following:

- What's important to remember is. . .
- I can't answer that question, but I can tell you. . .
- Let me put this in perspective. . .

The PIO's responses must be coherent, consistent, and helpful. For example, see the following:

- We will do all we can to help you to make responsible decisions for yourself and your loved ones.
- We will not engage in speculation.
- We may need to withhold information that may aid terrorists.
- We have survived attacks in the past and will survive this one.

7.20 LOCAL HOSPITAL ACTION GUIDE

The hospitals' primary responsibility is to provide medical care and treatment for people who have been injured or are suffering from radiation burns. To control an influx of "worried well," who could otherwise absorb resources needed to save lives, hospitals should request law enforcement to cordon off access and redirect the worried well to the area established by the RC to monitor and reassure them.

The local hospital is responsible for indicating where ambulances should deliver victims at the established location. Ambulance personnel should stay in their vehicle until they have been surveyed and released by a radiological assessor after transportation services are concluded.

In providing treatment, hospital staff should assume that the patient is contaminated. They also should coordinate with the law enforcement, a security teams, and nFEMT to provide protection and security for the hospital and preserve evidence by doing the following:

- Handling any unknown metal objects with a hemostat or forceps.
- Saving and labeling samples (smears of contamination, nasal smear, extracted tooth, hair and nails, purged bone pieces, etc.).
- Segregating possible or confirmed radiological waste for later analysis, if considered necessary by a member of the nFEMT.
- Taking reasonable steps to control the spread of contamination in the hospital and the emergency room.
- After discharging patients, and at the end of the emergency phase, cleaning up the area, following the dose control procedures established by the radiological assessor. No one is permitted to return to the area until cleared by the RA.

7.21 NATIONAL EOC ACTION GUIDE

The National Emergency Operations Center is activated at the IC's request, typically in cases of significant media or international attention. Its role is to coordinate national support to the local response and to support the IC. The functions the National EOC undertake include the following:

- Informing appropriate authorities that the IC is leading the response, and briefing them on their roles
- Ensuring that responses to the media are coordinated through the local PIO and that the national interface with the media is moved to the local vicinity as soon as possible
- Establishing a communication line between the IC and RA to ensure ongoing consultation and advice on dealing with the radiological hazard and getting the RA to the site by military transport if that will save transportation time
- Activating a designated national hospital

- Dispatching the national radiological assessment team and other resources as required and coordinating their arrival with the IC or RC at the scene
- Keeping the IC informed of relevant, up-to-date intelligence
- Taking action to mitigate the economic and psychological consequences of the disaster, including the following:
  1. Restricting national and international trade of potentially contaminated items until they have been assessed against international standards
  2. Addressing concerns about national and international movement of potentially contaminated people
  3. Informing the media of actions taken, in coordination with the PIO
  4. Taking steps, such as enhancing security, to reduce the likelihood of similar events
  5. In cooperation with the IC, responding to international inquiries and rumors
  6. Having a national authority notify the IAEA and authorities in other nations, if there are indications that other states or their citizens may be affected
  7. If necessary, requesting international assistance through the IAEA.

7.22 FIRST RESPONDER MONITOR ACTION GUIDE

The first responder monitor must be equipped and experienced to perform basic radiation monitoring. However, this is not a substitute for the radiological assessment performed by the RA or team. Therefore, the first responder monitor must consult with the RA or team by phone before they arrive and keep open lines of communication among the first responders, the IC, and the RA, especially during transit.

The first responder monitor performs operational checks of the instruments. If more than one instrument is available, they perform crosschecks among instruments to ensure consistent readings and confirm that gamma dose rate meters can measure from 0.1μ to 1 Sv/hr. In a clean place outside the inner cordoned area, one instrument should be stored for monitoring low-level contamination.

The monitor arranges for areas to be marked with day-glow spray paint where ambient dose rates are as follows:

- Greater than 100 mSv/hr (area where only life-saving actions should be performed, and time there should be limited to less than 30 minutes)
- Greater than 0.1 mSv/hr (boundary of inner cordoned area)

In addition, responsibilities include monitoring for gamma, beta and alpha radiation (as equipped), and immediately informing the radiological assessor/ team if alpha radiation is detected. The first responder monitor essentially plays a support role to the other response teams by screening public groups and locations (e.g., hospitals) to locate and isolate sources with ambient dose rates above 100 μSv/hr at least 1 m and by supporting the decontamination procedure of people and equipment. They also support the response contamination control area, the actions of law enforcement/security team and nFEMT, and the actions of the local hospital.

Finally, the monitor keeps records of people monitored and fully briefs the radiological assessor or team upon their arrival.

In the next chapter, we will examine step by step how the roles and responsibilities of first responders are put into action in the event of a radiological emergency.

CHAPTER 8

ACTION PLANS

8.1 ASSESS HAZARD AND ESTABLISH SECURITY AREA

The first responder who arrives from emergency services is responsible for assessing the hazard. First, he or she must determine whether a radiological threat exists. Indications of a possible radiological emergency are as follows:

- The confirmed or suspected presence of a bomb or explosive device designed to volatilize or scatter isotopes
- Credible threats or threatening messages
- A device that seems to be intended to spread contamination
- Signs of possible contamination (e.g., a spill)
- Gamma dose rates: > 100 μSv/hr at 1 m from object, or at 1 m above the ground
- Medical symptoms of radiation injuries (e.g., burns without an apparent cause)
- A building or area marked with the radiation symbol
- Neutron activation of a material
- Knowledge that a dangerous source is lost, stolen, damaged, in a fire, leaking, or potentially involved in a terrorist act or explosion

Radiation Safety: Protection and Management for Homeland Security and Emergency Response. By L. A. Burchfield

Indications of a dangerous source include the following:

- A heavy container with the radiation symbol
- Labels indicating that an item contains radioactive or fissile material
- Labels with relevant transport UN numbers or markings
- Device used for cancer treatment (teletherapy or brachytherapy)
- Radiography cameras or sources
- Well logging sources used in drilling operations

The radiological assessor will measure, assess, and verify whether a radiological hazard in fact exists and how serious it is. Until then, however, the first responder should establish an inner cordoned safety area with a clearly defined, visible, secure perimeter and, within that area, follow the personnel protection guidelines and public protection guidelines provided below.

8.2   PERSONNEL PROTECTION GUIDELINES

All responders must adhere to the following guidelines when responding to a radiological emergency, unless directed otherwise by a radiological assessor (female workers who may be pregnant must be excluded from emergency duties):

- Follow the standard safety procedures for your profession.
- Be visually identifiable and ensure you are recorded when going inside the inner cordoned area.
- Do not touch suspected radioactive items, including bomb fragments.
- Perform only lifesaving actions within 1 m of a suspected dangerous radioactive material or source or 100 m of a fire or explosion, unless equipped with respiratory protection.
- Minimize time spent within 10 m of a suspected dangerous radioactive material or source.
- Go upwind when dust or smoke is or may be dispersing radioactive contamination.
- Use respiratory protection equipment or cover mouth with a mask or handkerchief. Also, keep hands away from mouth, do not smoke, eat, or drink, and wash hands frequently.
- Use standard precautions, such as surgical gloves and masks, when treating or transporting contaminated people.

- Ensure your name and the activities you perform are recorded, for possible follow-up and dose reconstruction.
- Get monitored for radioactive contamination after being within the inner cordoned area. Shower and change clothing as soon as possible and discard contaminated outer garments.
- Once emergency operations have ended, follow the occupational radiation protection guidance of the radiological assessor in undertaking activities such as source recovery, clean-up, and waste disposal.

It is important to monitor the work areas as soon as possible to learn the gamma dose rate. As soon as the radiological assessor arrives on scene, they will monitor the area for other forms of radioactivity. If the ambient dose rate in a particular area is more than 100 mSv/hr, perform only lifesaving actions, limit total time there to less than 30 minutes, and do not enter an area with an ambient dose rate of more than 1.0 Sv/hr, unless directed by a radiological assessor. It is important to follow these safety rules even when using self-reading dosimeters, because these do not measure the dose from inhalation, ingestion, or skin contamination.

8.3 PUBLIC PROTECTION GUIDELINES

The Internal Commander (IC) or their designee is responsible for applying these guidelines whenever they respond to a radiological emergency where members of the public are involved. They should instruct members of the public who are within the inner cordoned area when first responders arrive to take the best available shelter and stay away from windows, until they can evacuate and to evacuate as promptly as possible. The public should also be warned not to handle possibly radioactive items, but instead to isolate them and identify them to a responder. The public should be instructed not to smoke, eat, drink, or place their hands near their mouth, and to wash hands, shower, and change clothes as soon as possible to avoid inadvertent ingestion.

After evacuation, the IC should do the following:

- Register evacuees
- Remind them to avoid inadvertent ingestion, if contamination is a major concern
- Monitor them for radiation, if the means are available
- If warranted and practical, conduct immediate decontamination, as described below

- Tell them where to go for more information and medical or radiological assessment
- Instruct them on the need, after leaving the scene, to shower and change clothes as soon as possible, place their possibly contaminated clothes in plastic bags, and separate them from other clothes. (They should not wash the possibly contaminated clothes in the home or send them to a laundry or cleaner.) In addition, they should listen for more instructions on where to get information and medical or radiological assessment.

Some members of the public may leave the inner cordoned area without being registered. Through the media, or other means appropriate for the community, they should be instructed to follow these public safety guidelines.

Members of the public outside the inner cordoned area may be at risk if contaminated smoke or dust is spreading from a fire or bomb. Via the media, instruct the public that people within about 1 km of the release point should do the following:

- Shelter in place
- Cut off any ventilation to outside air
- Cover all windows and doors with a plastic wrap and duct tape to prevent entrance of radioactive dust particles into ones home or apartment
- Remain inside their building during the atmospheric release
- Not eat any vegetables grown outside or drink runoff or rainwater
- Suspend all outside activities especially children playing parks on open soil
- Wash their hands with soap and water before eating
- Avoid dusty areas or activities that will generate dust
- Listen for and follow official instructions given via the media

8.4 PUBLIC REGISTRATION

The fire department is typically responsible for registering members of the public who may have been within the inner cordoned area but who do not require immediate medical treatment or transport. Treatment and transport of seriously injured people should not be delayed for registration, monitoring, or decontamination. A secure, sheltered public registration area should be established outside the inner cordoned area.

If terrorism or criminal activity is suspected, it is important to ensure that people are searched for weapons before they come to the public registration area, and that emergency workers are protected from potentially armed suspects.

Furthermore, uninjured individuals who were within the inner cordoned area should be instructed on public safety guidelines and should go to a public registration area where they can wait safely while being processed. If contamination is not suspected, they should be registered and released. If they may be contaminated (e.g., in the presence of potentially radioactive smoke, liquid, or dust) and arrangements for decontamination are in place, they should be sent for decontamination, provided this does not interfere with necessary first aid. If they may be contaminated and arrangements for decontamination are not in place, they should be released after they have undergone the following steps:

- Registered
- Instructed in how to avoid inadvertent ingestion
- Told to shower and change their clothes when possible, and to place their clothes in a plastic bag and set them aside
- Told to listen for and follow official instructions given over the media

8.5 MONITOR THE PUBLIC AND RESPONDERS

It is beneficial to monitor people for radiation contamination when a first responder monitor or radiological assessor is available, and when it is possible that people may have been contaminated. However, monitoring is not essential, and it is always of secondary importance to medical treatment.

Only qualified individuals should conduct monitoring. All monitors should be aware that some instruments can be overwhelmed by very high radiation levels and can show a low or zero reading in dangerous areas. They should perform the following operational check of the monitoring instruments in an area away from the scene:

- Check the battery.
- Confirm that the instrument can measure ambient dose rates in the range of local background (typically $0.05-0.2$ μSv/hr). The monitor should understand the units displayed and how ranges are changed.
- Open the beta window, if available.
- Wrap the instrument in a plastic bag, and allow for only the probe to be exposed. Tape the probe handle with duct tape to reduce cross-contamination and aid in decontamination of the instrument.

- Record the instrument number and the background level in an area not close to the scene.
- Keep one check instrument in a "clean area" and do not use it for routine monitoring.
- Using an instrument that can read at least 100 mSv/hr, approach the scene with the instrument switched on. Do not enter areas with ambient dose rates greater than 100 mSv/hr.
- If terrorism or criminal activity is suspected, ensure law enforcement searches people for weapons and dispersive devices before they are monitored.
- Establish a monitoring location in an area with ambient dose rates below 0.3 μSv/hr that is close to the decontamination area.

To identify and isolate objects with an ambient dose rate greater than 100 μSv/hr at 1 m before members of the public enter the monitoring area, screen them away from the monitoring area. Have them walk within 2 m of an instrument measuring in a range of 100 μSv/hr or more. Isolate identified objects with an ambient dose rate greater than 100 μSv/hr.

When monitoring, qualified individuals should:

- Wear gloves and protective clothing as available, and change gloves regularly.
- Follow personnel protection guidelines provided above.
- Periodically get monitored and, if contaminated more than 0.3 μSv/hr get decontaminated.
- Periodically confirm that the instrument is operational and not contaminated by verifying that it can measure background radiation. If it is contaminated, then replace the plastic bag, and recheck.
- Monitor peoples' hair, hands, pockets, dirty parts of clothes, feet, and face, holding the monitor approximately 5 cm (2 in) from the monitored surface.
- Record the results of this contamination survey.
- Advise people how to decontaminate, if necessary, and send them home.

8.6   PUBLIC DECONTAMINATION

Typically, the fire department will oversee the decontamination area serving people who do not need immediate medical treatment or transport. Seriously injured victims should bypass decontamination; they should simply remove their outer clothing, wrap them in a blanket, and tag or mark these victims as possibly contaminated.

If it is not possible to establish a decontamination area promptly, the public should be reminded to shower and change clothing and set it aside as soon as possible, and then these persons should be released.

The decontamination area should be established outside the inner cordoned area. This location should have security, protection from the weather, and controlled entrance and exit points, and it should be appropriate for the available resources and number of people to be decontaminated.

In the case of field decontamination for large numbers, facilities should be provided for people to wash their hands and face and to remove their outer clothing partly.

Full decontamination for small numbers should provide separate areas for males and females to take a shower and immediately obtain clean clothing. Water used for decontamination should be collected, if it can be done without delaying the decontamination.

In addition, blankets, clothing, and anything else that could be used to dress people who have removed their outer clothing should be acquired and receipts should be provided for contaminated items, which are double-bagged and tagged as contaminated.

During decontamination, families should be kept together, and adults should assist children or others needing help.

8.7 RESPONSE CONTAMINATION CONTROL

A member of the fire department is typically responsible for contamination control of responders. If there is an indication that an area may be contaminated by the presence of radioactive smoke, liquid, or dust, a response contamination control area should be established at the boundary of the inner cordoned area, with provision for the following:

- A controlled entrance and exit
- Logging in and out of the area
- Collection and storage of equipment used inside the inner cordoned area

For decontamination of equipment, a hose line should be used and the best practicable runoff control put in place to ensure that it does not affect other operational areas.

For decontamination of personnel, the same two steps listed above should be implemented, and facilities to change outer clothing and wash hands and face should be provided. Provisions should be in place to replace protective equipment (air supplies and filters) and to bag and control waste. (Response contamination control is also responsible for ensuring that first responders follow steps to optimize safety and control contamination.)

After entering the inner cordoned area, personnel should do the following:

- Cover instruments with plastic bags
- Log in (keep account of those in the area)
- Control the number of additional tools going into the area (if possible, use tools already there)

After leaving the inner cordoned area, one should do the following:

- Remove plastic cover from the instruments
- Leave instruments and equipment used inside the inner cordoned area for further use
- Receive monitoring and field decontamination
- Before leaving the scene, get a full decontamination or, if decontamination is not performed, remain isolated until showered and all clothing changed and bagged
- Log out

8.8   MONITORING AND DECONTAMINATION OF VEHICLES AND EQUIPMENT

Equipment and items that were inside the inner cordoned area, as well as the vehicles used to transport potentially contaminated victims, cannot be released for general use until monitored by a radiological assessor. This includes private vehicles and taxis. Typically, the fire department is responsible for monitoring and decontaminating vehicles and equipment.

An equipment monitoring and decontamination area, equipped with decontamination supplies (e.g., fire hoses, scrub brushes, and detergents), should be established on the boundary of the inner cordoned area where the background ambient dose rate is below 0.3 μSv/hr.

Equipment monitoring procedures (listed previously) should be followed. In addition, to ensure that any objects with an ambient dose rate more than 100 μSv/hr at 1 m are identified and isolated before members of the public enter the monitoring area, the public should be screened away from the monitoring area. Set up an instrument measuring in a range of 100 μSv/hr or more where they will walk within 100 m of it, and isolate identified objects with an ambient dose rate greater than 100 μSv/hr.

When monitoring vehicles and equipment, personnel should take the following precautions:

- Wear gloves and protective clothing as available, and change gloves regularly.
- Periodically confirm the instrument is operational and not contaminated by verifying that it can measure background. If contaminated, replace the plastic bag and recheck.
- Monitor items for gamma contamination by holding the monitor about 10 cm from the surface. If contamination levels are greater than 1 μSv/hr, decontaminate using fire hoses, scrub brushes, and detergents. Do not delay or interfere with the response to remove or replace contaminated filters, and resurvey the contaminated areas.

8.9 FIELD TRIAGE FOR MASS CASUALTIES

Typically, the fire department is among the first on the scene and takes responsibility for field triage until it is relieved by the EMS. The first step is to establish the triage and first aid area outside the inner cordoned area but within the outer cordoned area. Also, staff should consider using a flashing blue light to draw people toward the triage/first aid area.

Serious medical problems always have priority over radiological concerns. Those who can respond to a voice announcement to come to the gathering point probably can wait for medical attention.

In a mass casualty situation, people should be categorized as follows:

- Priority 1: need immediate treatment
- Priority 2: need early treatment
- Priority 3: can wait for treatment
- No actions: no need for treatment

Victims should be tagged with their medical conditions and category.

Responders should provide first aid as required and obtain an estimate on the number of victims the transport unit and hospital can handle. The transport unit and the receiving medical facilities should be informed on the nature of event, number of injured people, nature of injuries, and cases of suspected or confirmed contamination or radiation exposure.

Transportation of the injured must be arranged depending on the nature of their injuries. Life-threatening injuries should be transferred to the nearest hospital. Non-life-threatening injuries should be transferred to the secondary hospital out of the area or, for radiation-induced injuries, to the designated hospital.

To limit the spread of contamination, if there is an indication that people could be contaminated, the following steps should be taken:

- Victims with life-threatening injuries should be wrapped in blankets or sheets and transported to the hospital immediately.
- Those with non-life-threatening injuries and noninjured people should undergo field or full decontamination, as appropriate, or be advised how to decontaminate themselves at home.

CHAPTER 9

MEDICAL TREATMENT OF RADIOLOGICAL INJURIES

We have discussed what members of the military, health-care staff, and first responders can do to protect public and national safety in the case of nuclear or radiological emergency. Now we need to take a closer look at how radiation affects the health—both immediately and over time, physically and psychologically—and how lives can be saved through the advancements of technology and medical treatments.

After all, once diplomacy, determent, and defense fail, these developments are our best hope.

9.1 THE RADIOLOGICAL EFFECTS OF RDDs

The detonation of a radiological dispersion device RDD or improvised nuclear device (IND) causes many medical concerns, beginning with blast injuries and burns to those closest to the bombsite and acute radiation syndrome developing in those victims trapped near high gamma-radiation doses. The explosion also releases radioactive material into the air, which can cause localized radiation injuries if it comes into contact with the eyes and skin or if it enters a wound. The finer radioactive materials attached to particles or those that have been vaporized are more easily ingested or inhaled and can be more

Radiation Safety: Protection and Management for Homeland Security and Emergency Response. By L. A. Burchfield
Copyright © 2009 John Wiley & Sons, Inc.

widely dispersed, which causes major environmental contamination. In addition to these physical injuries, the whole event can result in widespread psychological trauma in those who were (or who believe themselves to have been) exposed.

In each case, medical treatments and procedures must counteract the damage that radiation does to the human body, from the psychological to the cellular levels.

9.2   RADIOACTIVITY AND ITS IMPACT ON THE BODY

When radioactivity is released into the atmosphere and absorbed into the body, one of four things will happen. First, the radioactive substance passes cleanly through the cells, which means that no damage was done. The second scenario is that, although the cell may have been damaged, it was able to renew or heal itself before replicating and passing the damage along to new cells. The third possibility is that the damage was reproduced and ingrained into new cellular structure. Finally, the cell itself may have been irreparably damaged or killed.

If either of the first two circumstances occurred, the body did not sustain permanent damage or injury. If, however, the cellular damage was passed on to new cells, then delayed effects of the radiation may manifest, such as cancer or genetically induced disease. No real time limit is predicted as to when these diseases may show; it could be months or decades after the initial exposure to radiation. Furthermore, even low-level doses of radiation may have a subsequent adverse effect on health, although latency periods and the severity of the disease will depend on the amount, type, and duration of radioactivity involved (as well as on issues of personal health, age, immunity, and initial treatment).

This type of slow-release cellular damage is perhaps the most common and treacherous side effect associated with radioactivity. It can result in increased cancer levels among people living near nuclear lagacy, incidents of thyroid disease, a weakening of the immune system, damage to the nervous system, possible genetic effects, and birth defects. However, the linkage between gradual or low-level radioactive exposure and subsequent disease is highly contested for a variety of reasons. The first are political. The second are scientific: Other factors (such as smoking, air pollution, and additional environmental aspects) can result in similar diagnoses. Also, not everyone who undergoes the exact same exposure suffers these negative consequences.

Nevertheless, the statistics are hard to deny. In an extreme situation such as Chernobyl, where childhood thyroid cancer was practically nonexistent, cases jumped over 200% in the months and years after the nuclear fallout. In the case of people living near the Nevada test sites, where the detonation of nuclear weaponry had been ongoing, it seemed that nearly three quarters of cancer patients diagnosed in the region had been previously exposed to high doses of radiation. Even 27 years after the Marshall Island testing, inhabitants and subsequent generations were still showing increased signs of thyroid disease and cancer.

The fourth scenario of radioactive exposure, in which cells are instantly killed, could be followed shortly by death from radiation poisoning, skin lesions, chronic vomiting, and so on. Examples of this would be the Japanese citizens who survived the initial impacts of the atomic bombs but died within days or weeks of detonation.

What also must be taken into account is that different types of radiation have different health effects. Rem are the units commonly used to measure the amount of any radioactivity that body tissues absorb and, of course, the more rems the worse. However, equal doses of radiation may not result in equal amounts of damage. For example, although alpha particles are the least penetrating once absorbed into the body, they inflict more internal harm than either beta or gamma radiation because of their size and electrical charge. (Thus, lower levels of uranium exposure can have a more damaging effect than higher doses of photons, or gamma radiation, found in X-rays.)

The International Commission on Radiological Protection, which consists of a board of radiation experts acting without governmental leanings, determined that the maximum dosage of radiation that a person can be exposed to in 1 year should not exceed five rem (the unit that determines at which levels certain types of radiation will have an effect, because, as we have discussed, equal dosages do not apply to each form of radioactivity). Although the cumulative effect of a five-rem dosage could cause damage, 1 year is considered enough time for the bodily tissue that absorbed the radiation to rebuild itself.

Even though that standard of rem safety was established in 1928, it is still in effect for radiation workers today. However, many doctors contest that number, and they argue that any absorbed dosage over one rem increases a person's risk of cancer 20-fold.

Although there are, as we have examined in previous chapters, many benefits to controlled uses of radioactivity, and the effects of long-term, low-level radiation are still in question, the adverse effects that large quantities of radiation have on our bodies in the long term remain undisputed.

At high dosages, exposure to radiation can result in a decrease in white blood cells, which causes the immune system to be unable to fight off infection; even in low dosages, radiation increases the risk of cancer. Therefore, first responders and medical teams should use some simple protective gear, which ranges from medical masks to air purifying respirators, as a barrier against airborne radioactive particles, even in a low-level radiological incident or an RDD event.

With or without some protective measures, members of the military, first responders, and civilians in the vicinity of radiological or IND attacks might not realize the effects on their health until later diagnoses disclose them or future symptoms occur. In a mass-casualty accident or as a form of terrorism, radiation can do far-reaching physical and psychological damage in addition to the immediate impact it has on the body.

9.3   SYMPTOMS AND SYNDROMES

After the accident at Chernobyl, thousands of cases were documented of what is known as uneven distribution of exposure because of shielding. If a victim was only partially protected from radiation, pockets of regenerative cells in blood-forming tissues could survive, despite the high dosages received in other parts of the body.

When this is the case, subsequent operations intended to save the patient's life, such as bone marrow transplants (which were especially common because bone marrow cells divide and regenerate rapidly, causing them to survive and pass on radioactive matter rather than die instantly like many cells), turned out to be cruelly unsuccessful, because the new bodily material was often rejected by the surviving tissue. Not enough of the victim's body had died to accept the transplant but not enough had survived to go on living without it.

Most Chernobyl victims were exposed to high levels of radiation that most likely would not occur from an RDD or IND attack. However, depending on radiation dosage, different life-threatening malfunctions occur in the body shortly after exposure; collectively, these malfunctions are known as acute radiation syndrome (ARS). For the sake of brevity here, we will examine three main categories of ARS that commonly appear after a nuclear incident, although these symptoms can take many forms. They are listed based on their occurrence from lowest to highest doses of radiation.

Hematopoietic symptoms may start to appear 2 weeks after detonation or a nuclear incident and, as the name suggests, affect blood-forming organ tissues. The radiation absorbed by the body and the damage done to these organs generally result in a decrease in the white blood cell count, which leads to decreased immunity, increased infection, and uncontrolled bleeding.

The second category of symptoms, gastrointestinal, can manifest within a week after high levels of radiation exposure. Although this dosage may be survivable, internally ingested radioactive materials can have the propensity to destroy intestinal lining, which causes excessive fluid loss and possibly a complete loss of the intestinal wall.

Neurovascular symptoms comprise the final category and can appear earlier than the other two, in as short a time as a day or two after high doses of radiation exposure, such as those suffered by victims nearby a radiological bombsite vicinity and first responders to mid- or high-level incidents. The presence of neurovascular symptoms means that irreversible damage has been done to the central nervous system, for which no treatment is available.

Although each of these categories is extremely serious in itself and can result in critical conditions or even death, more medical complications occur after nuclear or radiological incidents when radiation injuries combine with more immediate bodily damage sustained from the blast wave or burns from the nuclear thermal effect. These compounded injuries make a victim's chances for survival much slimmer—and therefore their emergency medical needs a much lower priority—than those suffering from either conventional impact wounds or even radiation absorption alone. Yet in the case of a nuclear explosion, it can be expected that up to 70% of medical emergencies would involve such combination injuries.

9.4 EMERGENCY ASSESSMENT

In any event that involves above average levels of radiation, it may be impossible to determine which, if any, long-term symptoms or diseases may develop as a result. In an emergency situation, that is not even the goal; treating apparent injuries and immediate casualties in the first few hours after exposure takes precedence over predicting long-term consequences. In that way, local hospitals and health-care facilities function like secondary decontamination (decon) and triage centers near nuclear blast sites or in locations with high concentrations of radiological dispersion.

Hospitals further away or trauma facilities prepared for tertiary care and reachable by emergency medical transport would be the appropriate places for some combined injury patients or those suffering from ARS to receive requisite surgery. Even so, candidates for more complicated surgical procedures must be screened and chosen carefully to conserve time and resources in an emergency situation with limited supplies and staff. Only those who can be treated within a day and a half of significant radiation exposure (and who have not suffered extensive compounded injuries) will be considered for surgical treatment.

To assess whether ensuing treatment will be forthcoming or even necessary, the primary step is to identify the radionuclides to which victims have been exposed; these radionuclides will often determine the kind of external or internal damage incurred. In fully equipped laboratories, proportional counters are the most typical devices used to determine alpha, beta, or gamma radiation absorption. However, these laboratories take some time to deliver accurate results.

In less than optimum circumstances, health-care personnel should still be capable of finding out this information with more limited radiation-detecting equipment, such as surface monitoring smears or portable hand-held radiation monitors. In this process, hospital staff simply "wand" the alpha/beta probe just a few millimeters above the patient. If a sterile field is required, sterile filter paper can be wiped across the skin or tissue surface then measured with a portable rate meter or scintillation counter that is keep nearby but outside the sterile field. From the results, medical professionals can quickly and easily determine whether a patient is contaminated with alpha-emitting radioisotopes (from polonium, uranium, or plutonium, for example) or beta emitters (such as radioactive strontium or cesium).

More advanced bioassay radiation testing can assess the rate at which lymphocyte counts drop, which reveals the radiation dosage absorbed by the body. This test can be administered through blood samples from a finger prick and therefore can be performed even by emergency personnel with relatively little experience. However, because comparison samples must be taken, the test should be administered every 6 hours or at the very least once a day; thus, both a stable medical environment and almost immediate testing after initial radiation exposure is required for the most accurate result readings and for the most effective follow-up treatment.

Following a radiological event, there will potentially be hundreds to thousands of people in need of testing—and provisions must be made for the thousands more who *want* to be tested for contamination. Even though it will be difficult to determine the amount of radiation exposure for each victim involved in a mass-casualty disaster because of time and resource constraints, some short-term signs and symptoms give an indication of the dosage received and can therefore assist in diagnosing internal damage.

9.5 SIGNS OF DANGEROUS RADIATION DOSAGES

In a situation with a large number of victims, sometimes a cursory diagnostic screening can be made based on symptoms exhibited shortly after radiation exposure. Although this diagnosis may not give an exact assessment of internal damage, it can provide enough information to categorize a patient as having "unlikely, probable, or severe" radiation injury, and thus medical staff determine what type of care, if any, can mitigate it.

One sign of having received potentially life-threatening doses of whole-body gamma radiation is a tingling or lightly burning sensation of the skin, even though no wounds or burns exist (alpha particles cannot penetrate the body if the skin is intact). Rising body temperature might also be related to high dosages; the sooner the body temperature increases, in general the more elevated the dose level may be.

If the skin is peeling or flaking, the patient may have come into external contact with high doses of beta particles, which were allowed to remain for more than an hour (if decon does not take place, beta burns may occur). If high external doses were received in a localized area on an extremity, amputation may be the most efficient and immediate form of treatment.

A patient may experience fatigue and nausea from even low levels of radiation, which could be contributed to the traumatic experience as much as actual radiation injury. However, severe and immediate vomiting indicates the ingestion or inhalation of high doses of radiation; if it continues or diarrhea ensues, then the patient may be beyond the help of medical treatments. In addition, the occurrence of respiratory, metabolic and neurological symptoms without the appearance of conventional injuries may indicate terminal radiation damage.

How the immediate or fallout radiation was received—whether through ingestion, inhalation, or wound contamination/skin absorption—can also convey information about injury and possible treatment. Of these, inhalation is the worst-case scenario. Fine particles are the most easily absorbed by the lungs, although a quarter of these may be expelled by simple exhalation; the other three quarters, however, will be absorbed in the body and circulate themselves among internal compartments, starting from the trachea, moving to the bronchial tree within a few hours (where lethal amounts of absorbable alpha emitting isotopes may remain in the lungs for months or years), then to the digestive and, finally, gastrointestinal tracts.

With treatment for internal contamination, time is of the essence. Effective care should begin within hours of exposure to keep spreading to a minimum, especially in cells that replicate rapidly (although that is not always a possibility in emergency situations). Radiation symptoms will appear in stages, and their severity and duration correspond to dosages received: *prodromal* symptoms can occur within a few hours to about 4 days after exposure; a *latent* stage brings symptom relief that may last about a month but is followed by *manifest* illness, during which immunity is most compromised. After this final stage, chances for survival increase greatly. Therefore, the treatment a patient receives from initial exposure throughout the first 3 months is crucial in recovery from radiological injuries.

In an emergency situation, however, that kind of care is not always possible. The foremost focus is on basic life support that addresses conventional, life-threatening wounds in patients who fall into the "unlikely" category of having internal radiation injuries. In probable cases of radiation injury, it is important that ventilation and circulation are first kept functioning for improved chances of survival, and that risks of infection are kept to a minimum because immunity is compromised. Concerns about severe radiation absorption sustained by a patient unfortunately come last in an emergency situation—even though several treatments are available.

9.6 TREATMENTS FOR RADIATION EXPOSURE

In 2004, the U.S. Department of Health and Human Services began work in conjunction with the National Institute of Allergy and Infectious Diseases (NIAID) and the National Institutes of Health to research and develop medical countermeasures against radiological attacks from terrorists. Before then, many of these pharmaceuticals were cleared at the federal level only for military purposes, not civilian usage. However, as the threat of RDDs and INDs increases, it has become a federal priority to acquire and stockpile medical countermeasures for the general public that will prevent bodily tissue from absorbing or reacting to large amounts of radiation in cases of national emergency. For such purposes, the focus is on four main types of pharmaceuticals.

Blocking agents are used to decrease the absorption of radioisotopes by blocking their integration into active cells. In this way, fewer intercellular ionizations be created and the radiosotopes will be expelled from the body. One radioprotectant, Amifostine, is the first blocking agent to have already been approved by the Food and Drug Administration. Its active ingredient is a free radical that prevents radioactive substances from entering cell membranes and DNA molecules. Testing has shown that Amifostine decreases cell death and the chances of both mutagenesis and carcinogenesis in animals and cell systems.

Diluting agents flood the body with stable isotopes of the same element, which decreases the chances for absorption of radioactive isotopes.

Mobilizing agents increase the cells' regeneration process, which causes radioisotopes to be released more quickly from internal tissues.

Chelating agents, which we have touched on briefly before, bind strongly together with some metallic radioactive elements, which forms stable substances that can be more easily excreted from the body.

All of these pharmaceuticals are most effective when taken immediately, within 2 hours of radiation exposure, before the radioactive materials have had a chance to insinuate themselves within the cells (chelating agents, for example, cannot pass into cell membranes). However, some of these treatments, such as mobilizing agents, retain their efficacy for up to 2 weeks after exposure.

In addition, there are other, nonpharmaceutical options for treatment of radiation exposure. Sodium bicarbonate (which is fairly common in the form of baking soda) can be taken as a limited countermeasure to certain types of uranium, an agent often used in RDDs or INDs. Potassium iodide can be taken orally if a radioactive iodine substance is used as a contaminant. Magnesium sulfate will form compounds with radium, which can then be excreted. Even regular, over-the-counter antacids will help to reduce gastrointestinal absorption of ingested radionuclides (ones that contain aluminum can reduce strontium absorption by half to 85%).

Cytokines, which are naturally occurring types of protein, are particularly useful to treat bone marrow maladies because they increase the proliferation of marrow cells and cause them to diversify rather than recreate the radiated cells. Certain types of cytokines bind to the surface of hematopoietic receptor cells, which stimulates the generation and differentiation of other cells and inactivates the ones that have absorbed radiation. Because cytokines occur naturally, is a sufficient supply is available for use in mass casualty radiological events.

9.7 POST-RADIATION PROCEDURES

The timely treatment of victims suffering from internal radiation contamination will help to reduce the amount of radiation that is absorbed in the body, in this way also decreasing the risks of long-term consequences, such as cancer and genetic defects. As indicated in the pharmaceutical treatments, the two ways to achieve radiation reduction are by blocking the absorption of radionuclides and encouraging their rapid excretion.

A variety of procedures is available to help decontaminate the respiratory and gastrointestinal tracts, both of which are prime targets for the absorption of radioactive laden particles. Of course, to determine which procedure is most appropriate, the radioactive dose and toxicity of the sources must be taken into account, as well as the risk and side effects associated with the treatment itself. However, the advantage is that most of these procedures can be placed into immediate effect.

Gastric lavage (using a stomach pump and a slightly saline solution) will empty the stomach of ingested radioactive materials. It is most effective when performed within 2 hours of exposure to large dosages and should not be performed more than twice.

If the amount of radioactivity ingested is very large, cathartics and enemas can reduce dosages by encouraging quick expulsion, which decreases the chance for absorption. Enemas that involve phosphate soda can clean out the colon within minutes; oral laxatives or suppositories take longer but are less labor intensive.

Pulmonary lavage is a procedure that can be used in rare instances when extremely high doses of insoluble radionuclides are inhaled or ingested;

although the procedure itself is a bit risky, leaving large amounts of radioactive isotopes in the heart could lead to major pulmonary complications.

For each of these procedures, the cost is low and the process is relatively simple; however, they are not part of the triage procedure in cases of emergency with mass casualties because they require a lot of medical assistance. For example, a four-person medical team could perform these methods of decontamination on only about half a dozen patients per hour, compared with the 200 who go through gross decon in the same time frame.

A longer term procedure that targets hematopoietic syndromes after low- to mid-dosage radiation exposure, such as that experienced by many victims of nuclear or radiological accidents, can increase the number of platelets in the blood within a few weeks. The treatment involves the harvesting of platelets, which are cryogenically stored and later reinfused into the body, and it was performed successfully on a large number of Chernobyl patients.

Finally, stem cell transplants also can increase the hematopoietic cells in bone marrow, without as much trouble with the body's rejecting the new material that bone marrow transplants often encounter.

Even after immediate or more time-consuming medical procedures, however, there is still a chance that even though the body can repair itself, the mind may suffer irreparable traumatic damage from radiological events.

9.8 PSYCHOLOGICAL SIDE EFFECTS

During World War II, estimates of psychological casualties ranged from 18% to 40% and comprised the largest cause of weakened military forces. It can be assumed that some of these cases were the result of witnessing the devastation and radiological aftermath of the atomic bomb.

At that time, Brigadier General James Cooney reported his concern that his soldiers would not be able to function well in nuclear warfare for fear that radiation would bring about their "immediate and mysterious injury or death." In any event that involves radiation (including nuclear warfare and accidents, INDs or RDDs), those same fears still persist today.

Because symptoms of radiation exposure can manifest in years to come, victims often feel vulnerable, anxious, and uncertain about their futures; they entertain worst-case health scenarios that may carry over to their potential offspring and the contamination of the environment. Even in the long term, nuclear and radiological fallout brings with it anxiety about the potential to annihilate humankind.

Psychoses, neuroses, psychosomatic symptoms, and posttraumatic stress disorders often occur after life-threatening natural and man-made disasters—and will likely appear in a large percentage of any population that experiences even a small-scale nuclear or radiological attack. Many victims will continue to suffer from trauma, reliving and fixating on the event or feeling anxiety over the possibility of other external threats occurring. Those suffering from posttraumatic stress disorder will startle easily and experience irritability and strong reactions, as well as exhibiting abnormalities in their personalities and dreams.

Trying to predict which psychological side effects may manifest in the general public after a radiological event is often more difficult than predicting the appearance of long-term health effects. Depression and bereavement, interpersonal conflict, troubled sleep, difficulty concentrating, feelings of helplessness, increased smoking, alcohol and drug addiction, paranoia, and other signs of psychological distress will be widespread, alongside symptoms that may be the result of physical illness or psychosomatic manifestations.

In an emergency event, hospitals and medical facilities already besieged with victims will be flooded with others seeking care for possible exposure, which will only add to the chaos. Some may actually be suffering from acute radiation sickness, whereas others will show phantom symptoms that are not physically attributable to the event. A conservative estimate is that only one out of four patients who want to be evaluated will need medical treatment. Even years after the event, symptoms and illnesses will be wrongly attributed to radiation.

However, a real connection exists between the physical impact that radiation has on the nervous tissue and psychological changes that occur as a result. Studies undertaken 5 years after the atomic bombs were dropped in Japan and a few years after the Chernobyl nuclear meltdown show that memory and intellectual capacity decreased in victims of acute radiation sickness.

9.9 PSYCHOLOGICAL FIRST AID

Like radiological countermeasures that work best when administered immediately, certain psychological intervention provided in the first hours and days after a traumatic event are often more effective. Perhaps the most important step in patients' psychological well-being is actual medical attention. After that, providing a feeling of safety and shelter, even in a hospital steeped in pandemonium amidst an emergency, is essential. Other short-term factors include explaining medical services and support to the victims, keeping them informed of the situation by dispelling misinformation about the effects of radiation and detailing the course of recovery, and reuniting them with or helping them locate family.

In the weeks after a radiological attack or event, psychological therapy or treatment is still necessary. Patients should be encouraged to rest and return to normal routines; they should avoid or decrease their intake of reminders about the event, which includes overexposure to media coverage, disturbing images, and so on. Patients also should reestablish social and community bonds (through organizations, religious institutions, and the like) and communicate openly with family and friends, which can prompt discussion of fears and detect radical changes in personality.

9.10 TREATING TERROR

The thought of a radioactive device exploding strikes fear into most people's hearts. Although the physical impact may be similar to that of a conventional bomb, the psychological fallout is not even close. For that reason, they are the tools of choice for terrorists, whose aim is more to damage infrastructure, economics, and national psyche than to reach a certain body count.

Because confusion and a lack of expert agreement increases public fear, it is important that the responsibilities of the military, medical facilities, and first responders (laid out in the previous chapters) are clear and their roles in a radiological emergency are carried out clearly and concisely according to specification. Leadership, cohesiveness, and stable group structure play a vital and necessary part in preserving civil order and an individual's psychological health.

Transparency in federal information is also important. It has been shown that in combat, participants will overestimate the inherent danger and more likely fall victim to false rumors and hysteria if they are not briefed on the facts; the same is true for civilians under attack or in crisis situations.

With the global atmosphere today, while Americans brace themselves for the "next" 9/11 and plans for nuclear warheads are smuggled into rogue states, radiological attacks and incidents will most likely be inevitable. National and international security measures are firmly in place to guard against these scenarios. However, on an individual level, the best way to combat terrorism is to keep our deep-seated fears about radiation from turning into full-blown terror. Armed with information, we can dispel the myths and science-fiction specter of radiation to which we have been exposed for too long.

CHAPTER 10

CLEANUP AND DECONTAMINATION AFTER A RADIOLOGICAL INCIDENT

A radiological terrorist attack will most likely be a greater threat to buildings, infrastructure, and the environment than to people. After all, people are mobile, but buildings are not. This simple fact leads to perhaps the most daunting task after a radiological terrorist attack—cleanup and decontamination.

Although the immediate vicinity of a radiological terrorist attack will likely result in very high dose rates, the good news is that most of this activity will be contained (initially) in a relatively small area. The bad news is that many of the typical radioactive materials that might be used in a radiological dispersion device (RDD) may have very long half-lives. Coupled with rain and wind, this fact can make the cleanup from a radiological or nuclear incident difficult and challenging. This chapter reviews specific challenges and concepts in regard to the cleanup phase of a radiological incident.

10.1 DIFFERENCES BETWEEN CHEMICAL, BIOLOGICAL, AND RADIOLOGICAL

Radioactive isotopes are different from both chemical and biological hazards because the latter can be decomposed (chemical) or disinfected (biological), whereas the former has no physical or chemical means of altering its

Radiation Safety: Protection and Management for Homeland Security and Emergency Response. By L. A. Burchfield
Copyright © 2009 John Wiley & Sons, Inc.

half-life (other than using high-energy nuclear activation—which would not be practical for use during a radiological event). Thus, many isotopes that may be used in an RDD have very long half-lives (See Appendix E). However, if a short-lived isotope were to be used (although not likely), its impact could be minimized by simply allowing it to decay away. If an isotope undergoes 6 half-lives, it will only contain 1.6% of the original activity, and after 10 half-lives, it will contain a mere 0.1% of the original activities. This strategy would be effective with an isotope that has a half-life of days or perhaps weeks. However, it would not be practical solution with a half-life of say 30 years as is the case with cesium-137.

10.2   DECONTAMINATION DIFFERENCES FOR FALLOUT AND A RDD

During the Cold War, much expense and effort was put forward to protect the country from nuclear fallout. Survival from these types of incidents consisted almost entirely in the form of fallout shelters (stocked with food and water). In fact, in the 1950s, it was almost a status symbol to have your own "backyard" fallout shelter. Also, many large cities relied on public shelters with a high capacity for retreat from a potential nuclear confrontation using atomic bombs.

If we examine the differences between nuclear fallout and contamination from an RDD, we find significant differences. In nuclear fallout, the particle size ranges from 100 to 200 microns. Additionally, because these particles were born in the fireball of a nuclear weapon, they form high-fired oxides similar to the glaze on pottery and therefore tend to be relatively inert to chemical weathering. However, radiological contaminants from a "dirty bomb" or RDD may consist of very fine particles (even submicron size) or they may exist as aerosols or liquids. Moreover, contaminants from an RDD may consist of different radioisotopes that have different affinities for man-made surfaces, such as buildings, rooftops, or pavement, which makes the decontamination process from an RDD much more difficult than would be expected from fallout the detonation of a nuclear weapon. Also, as previously stated, radioactive contamination can not be destroyed, and the only thing one can do is to remove it from one surface and move it to a radiological burial site. In short, move it from one spot to another.

Decontamination of surfaces will perhaps present one of the biggest challenges depending on what type of radionuclide is "fixed" or attached to the surface. For example, the cesium ion is in the same family of elements as sodium and potassium (the alkali metals). Because sodium and potassium are very mobile in the environment, one would expect cesium to have the same properties. However, that is not the case. Cesium has an ion size of roughly

2.35 Å (1 Å $= 1 \times 10^{10}$ meters). It just so happens that this is the perfect size to be trapped in the silicate matrix of sand. Because sand is a very ubiquitous material used to construct buildings, sidewalks, and roadways, many surfaces will therefore readily absorb radioactive cesium-137, which provides a difficult path for cleanup. In fact, soil that has not been disturbed since the 1960s contains a layer of cesium-137 (from open-air testing of atomic bombs that spread radioactive fallout all over the planet) that is still easily identifiable today. Therefore, a soluble solution of cesium-137 will penetrate cement surface up to 5 mm deep and will create a difficult scenario for removal.

Some surfaces are easily cleaned or decontaminated. Such surfaces include painted, glass, ceramic, and enamel plates or any smooth nonporous material. However, materials such as bricks, mortar, or concrete present complicated scenarios because of their porosity and trapping ability. What this means fundamentally is that if you have road or building materials one can "wash off" or mechanically remove the first layer, although standard decontamination techniques will reduce the activity, they will not in most cases completely remove all contamination. As a result, decisions will have to be made as to how good is good enough and at what cost. These very difficult questions cannot and will not be ascertained prior to a radiological event. It will therefore, take a concerted effort on the part of many dedicated (and perhaps brave) individuals to remove the source of the problem effectively.

10.3 WHO WILL BE IN CHARGE OF CLEANUP AND DECONTAMINATION?

In August 2008, the Department of Homeland Security (DHS) issued *Planning Guidance and Recovery Following Radiological Dispersal Devices (RDD) and Improvised Nuclear Device (IND) Incidents.* This guidance is intended for federal, state, and local governments as well as emergency management personnel and the general public for developing planned recovery from radiological events (See Appendix F).

The guidance recommends protective action guides (PAGs) to support decisions about actions that should be taken to protect the public and emergency workers when responding to or recovering from an RDD or IND incident. This guidance also outlines a process to implement the recommendation and discusses existing operational guidelines that should be useful in the implementation of the PAGs and other response actions. The guidance also encourages federal, state, and local emergency personnel to implement these guidelines to develop specific operational plans and response protocols for protection of emergency workers responding to catastrophic incidents that involve high levels of radiation and/or radioactive contamination.

After immediate lifesaving measures have been made, the principle oversight for cleanup and decontamination in the United States will fall primarily under the auspices of the Environmental Protection Agency (EPA). The number of scenarios under which a radiological event will occur are too many and too complex for one to make any accurate prediction. The time of the event, location, type of radiological material used, size and type of weapon(s), amount of activity, means of dispersal, and types of facilities and infrastructure affected all have a bearing on how a cleanup will take place. Another quandary will also be to determine how good is good enough while affecting the decontamination process. The good news in this respect is that both the EPA and the Nuclear Regular Commission (NRC) already have guidelines in place for affecting superfund cleanups (ala EPA) and for the decontamination and decommissioning of nuclear facilities (ala NRC). The bad news is that each agency has or sets different cleanup criteria: 15 mrem per year above background radiation levels for the EPA, whereas the NRC has consistently enforced a standard of 25 mrem per year above background levels of radiation. To the casual reader, this difference may not seem like much; however, these levels are enormous in terms of the money, manpower, and resources that will be needed to affect radiological cleanup to these levels. Coupled with the fact that the average individual in the United States receives an annual dose of 360 mrem from natural and man-made radioactive sources, this fact can make such goals (esp. 15 mrem) nearly impossible or highly impractical. In essence, the cure could be worse than the cause, which is why the federal government has not set such limits for a radiological disaster.

10.4 RADIOLOGICAL CLEANUP OVERVIEW AND OBJECTIVES

According to the DHS August 2008 *Planning Guidance*, no numerical cleanup values are explicitly defined. The consensus of the federal government was that a numerical value would restrict the flexibility needed by state, local, and federal governments. Instead, the federal government has selected a framework in which a consensus is met through the use of an advisory group and a risk management approach. This approach does not attempt to provide detailed requirements to local officials. Instead, it assumes those details will be provided in state- and local-level planning documents, which address radiological terrorist events. The good news for the cleanup phase is that decision makers will have more time and information. In fact, the cleanup phase is no longer an emergency response; instead, it can be viewed in terms of site recovery and restoration.

In developing guidance planning, DHS has enlisted the experience from existing programs such as the EPA's Superfund program and the NRC's decontamination and decommissioning (to terminate a nuclear power plant license) as well as other national and international recommendations that may be useful in executing an effective cleanup following an RDD or IND incident. The DHS guidance also allows consideration and incorporation, as appropriate, of any or all of the existing environmental program elements.

Relevant site-specific procedures should include both qualitative (what is present) and qualitative assessments (how much is present) at each stage of the cleanup process. Included among the major components of the cleanup process are: (1) decision making, (2) initial scoping, (3) stakeholder outreach, (4) evaluation of cleanup options, and (5) implementation of selected cleanup options.

10.5 RADIOLOGICAL CLEANUP DECISION MAKING

For decision making (relative to cleanup) to be effective there must be stakeholder participation. At a minimum, decision making may require compromise and perhaps some negotiations. These compromises must be balanced with an informed risk review and analysis. In other words, risks will need to minimized and at the same time must affect practical measures in removal of radioactive contamination and restoring public access or release of personal property. In some cases, win–win solutions that allow divergent views to achieve their primary goals may be afforded. However, perhaps most decision making will require decision makers to compromise between potential long-term health risks (from low levels of exposure to radiation) and the need to restore access and use of facilities and infrastructure.

In many cases, the fundamental principle for decision making will hinge on abating public fears and restoring public confidence as well as the local economy. Long-term economic consequences, moreover, could be very significant if affected areas included major commercial or industrial sites and could not be readily restored to public use. For example, suppose that a major city had a radiological release of 15 mrem (0.015 rem) that covered 40 city blocks or one square mile. According to the EPA's cleanup guidelines, this risk level corresponds to one death to cancer out of a population of 10,000 over a 40-year exposure period. To some, this will be an acceptable risk to others—fear will dictate instead. Now, what if such a scenario were to occur near the U.S. Capitol? Would such levels be tolerated? And how "clean" is clean enough? Depending on the extent of contamination along with the desired cleanup levels, affected areas could be closed off for months or even years.

Losses in trade and commerce (and potentially property values) could range in the billions of dollars. David Pierson of the *LA Times* reported that researchers at the University of Southern California's Center for Risk and Economic Analysis of Terrorist events (CREATE) estimated that the total economic loss from an incident which hypothetically shut down the ports at Los Angles and Long Beach would cost as much as $34 billion dollars. Additionally, these losses would be compounded by the widespread fear and panic that would ensue from a radiological terrorist attack.

Decontamination levels will have to be well thought out and well managed. The problem with this concept, however, is that there is much interagency debate about what constitutes a reasonable radiological cleanup level, as well as what are real health effects with exposure to low levels of radiation. A very conservative approach has been to make the exposure levels as low as achievable. This approach is deemed the Linear No Threshold Limit (LNT) model. Scientists who support this model believe in the conservative assumption that even low levels of radiation exposure carry a quantifiable risk of cancer. Although this model is simple to apply in regulatory statutes, the actual scientific validity is contested by many scientists. In general, these scientists cite the lack of conclusive evidence of radiation effects at levels below 5 to 10 rem. The reason for this controversy is the lack of long-term studies coupled with the fact that numerous vectors in our environment can also cause cancer, which compounds the problem. For planners and decision makers, the activity selected within a radiological event will most likely occur somewhere between what we are exposed to from natural background levels (360 mrem or .36 rem) to perhaps a factor 10 times that amount (3600 mrem or 3.6 rem).

If the mantra from a radiological cleanup perspective becomes "how low can you go," then the mantra from an economic cost perspective will become "how much can we afford to spend." In the end, compromise will no doubt play an important role in the decision-making process.

10.6   INITIAL CLEANUP SCOPING

During the scoping phase of a radiological cleanup the following steps will need to be considered.

1. Determine what types of isotopes are present and at what activity levels. Additionally supporting chemical and physical evidence will be ascertained.

2. What chemical form is the radioactive material in? Also, one must determine whether it is a solid, liquid, or a highly unlikely gas (or volatile substance such as polonium or radioiodine).

These initial scoping actions will be critical in assisting decision makers on the most likely path for cleanup.

Senior decision makers will integrate all available information into a map for assessing first what needs cleanup and second what are the priorities.

10.7 STAKEHOLDER OUTREACH AND STAKEHOLDER WORKING GROUP

Stakeholders are selected federal, state, and local representatives; local non-government representatives; and local/regional business professionals. The exact makeup of the stakeholder working group will depend on circumstances surrounding who is affected by the radiological event and who will derive benefit from restorative measures. It will be important for the incident commander (IC) and other senior officials to enlist the support of the public immediately following a radiological event. Stakeholder outreach will be important for establishing lines of communication and more importantly as means of calming fear.

A stakeholder working group should be convened as soon as practical after the radiological event. This meeting would normally happen within days of the incident. How and where the stakeholder working group will meet will be dictated mainly by circumstances and will be coordinated with the public information officer to work with the group and thereby establish a liaison for public input to the entire process. The stakeholder working group will meet to review information and to provide input to the process. The level of detailed involvement in the working group will be defined and shaped by the circumstances, the number of people affected, the IC, and the stakeholder working group itself. The entire effort will be to restore normalcy as efficiently as possible, and the stakeholder working group will provide an invaluable communication link as well as a means of relieving fears and restoring calm.

10.8 EVALUATION OF CLEANUP OPTIONS

A technical working group will be convened as soon after the radiological incident as possible, most likely with days of the event. This group provides multiagency and multidisciplined scientist and engineers that will address the technical aspects of bringing about a safe and effective removal of radioactive materials present after an RDD or IND release. The technical working group will include selected scientists and engineers from federal, state, local, and private sector subject matter experts. The exact mix of technical experts selected will hinge on specifics of the radiological event. One group in particular will play a key role—radiochemists. Radiochemists are chemists that specialize in the chemical separation and analysis of all radioactive materials. Information about the science of radiochemistry can be found by going to the Radiochemistry Society website at www.radiochemistry.org.

The technical working group will review analytical data and provide solutions on the most effective means of release of the radiological event site back to the public. Most likely, this group will recommend a graded approach to cleanup. Common sense dictates that simple decontamination techniques will be deployed first, whereas deploying more costly and more stringent measures will be deployed on isolated "hot spots." Other aspects that will also have to be kept in mind are risks to personnel that affect the decontamination and cleanup, analysis of regulatory needs, as well as considerations of harm that the cleanup process itself will do to property or the environment.

10.9 SPECIFIC GUIDELINES FOR CLEANUP AND DECONTAMINATION

Essentially five major strategies can be used for decontamination and cleanup after a radiological incident as follows: (1) do nothing, (2) physical removal, (3) physical entrapment, (4) removal using chemical processes, and (5) isotope dilution. Each strategy has its benefits and weaknesses. Each needs to be considered carefully when formulating an overall strategy, and most are not mutually exclusive from one another and may be used in combination with one another. It is this combined strategy approach that offers a graded approach and allows for perhaps the most efficient means of decontamination success. For example, the physical removal processes may first deployed over a large range of areas and then smaller "hotspots" may be dealt with effectively on a smaller scale with a more aggressive approach.

10.10 THE "DO NOTHING" STRATEGY

The "do nothing" approach is as simple as it implies—do nothing. If the isotopes from an RDD have very short half-lives, then the most effective approach will be to allow the isotopes to decay. The rule is after an isotope goes through 6 half-lives, its activity level will be only at approximately 1.6% of the original activity. At 10 half-lives, there will only be 0.1% of the original activity. This approach will only be practical if the isotopes half-life does not exceed roughly 1 to 2 months. Of course, this also depends on not only which isotope is in question but also the original amount of radioactivity present.

10.11 PHYSICAL REMOVAL STRATEGY

Some radioactive materials have a tendency to embed themselves in porous surfaces. For example, cesium-137 is a 30-year beta/gamma emitter that has a propensity to "wedge" itself into porous materials that contain high amounts of silicates (concrete, brinks, roadways, sidewalks, roofs, building facades, etc.). The reason lies in the fact that the cesium ion size is just right to be physically trapped inside silicate matrices. Physical removal will consist of using physical force to remove radioisotopes from such surfaces. This action would include simple processes such as washing and trapping the runoff to the more aggressive process of grinding or physical demolition. Again, with such measures, a graded approach will be the most cost effective. For example, a street sweeper may be deployed to affect initial cleanup over large areas. This effort would also be supplemented with hand-held sprayers to affect areas where a street sweeper could not reach. After these simple efforts have been deployed and redeployed if necessary, the remaining radioactivity may have to be physically removed through sand blasting and grinding. One such technique that has proven to be particularly useful in removing radio-activity from a limited area uses "sand-blasting" with frozen CO_2 pellets. In general, physical removal processes can provide an effective means of removal of radioactivity; however, such activities can also be both time con-suming and costly, and care will have to be taken to assure that such activities are done in a safe and effective manner. For example, grinding processes would have to be controlled in such a manner to prevent the inhalation of dust. Physical removal processes will most likely be deployed to affect decon-tamination over large areas.

10.12 PHYSICAL ENTRAPMENT STRATEGY

Some isotopes only present a problem if they enter the body. In particular, iso-topes that emit alpha particles are a good candidate for physical entrapment. Physical entrapment means that another layer of material is added over a surface. Such materials include (but are not limited to) paint, plaster, plastics, cement, and so on. The idea behind this strategy would be to provide a means of "permanently" fixing or binding the contamination in such a manner that it will no longer be mobile. Perhaps the greatest example of this strategy occurred with the use of concrete to entomb the Chernobyl reactor. Another side to this strategy would be to use this as "temporary" means of holding or "locking" down an isotope so that it may be removed later and at leisure. A good example of this would be pavement sidewalks or roadways. Even if the "fixed" isotope was a gamma emitter, the dose to the public might be greatly minimized simply by the limited amount of time a motorist may spend over the entombed "hotspot."

10.13   CHEMICAL DECONTAMINATION STRATEGY

Chemical decontamination offers a more effective means of decontamination than physical decontamination can provide. Additionally, chemical decontamination offers a wider variety of chemicals that might be deployed.

To formulate a simplified chemical decontamination strategy, it will be necessary to understand some fundamental principles of chemistry. First, a chemical strategy needs to be based on what type of radioisotope needs to be removed from a surface. Elements can be classified as metals and nonmetals. Metals form cations (positive ions), and nonmetals form anions (negative ions). It turns out that most of the potential radionuclides that may be used in an RDD are metals rather than nonmetals. Perhaps the most significant exception to this rule would be radioactive iodine, which we will discuss later.

Another simple concept that needs to be understood by decision makers and those that affect cleanup is the concept of chelation and the ability to form complexes in solution. Only certain elements readily form complexes in solution, which include the transition elements (element in the third column to the twelfth column in the Periodic Table), as well as the lanthanides and actinides (elements listed in the two separated rows at the bottom of the periodic chart). These primary elements form complexes in solution. A complex is very important when chemical decontamination is deployed because it is the primary mechanism through which a radioactive contaminant that is fixed to a surface can be made soluble in an aqueous liquid. Perhaps the simplest display that everyone is familiar with is with the use of soap and water (actually two mechanisms are at work with soap and water—one involves the physical removal of small particles, and the other involves making the radioactive isotope soluble in water). Making the radioactive isotope actually dissolve in water (aqueous media) provides a power tool for radioactive decontamination.

On the positive side, some chemical decontamination strategies can be more aggressive and have less of an impact on structures and surfaces than say physical grinding. Also, chemical decontamination offers a wide variety of strategies that range from the very mild, nondestructive reagents to strong acids that will destroy the top layers of a surface. For example, perhaps the simplest strategy that is almost universal would be to use soap and water. Soap forms micelles that are effective at removing or surrounding grease and oils and can create an emulsion or water-soluble phase. Next, this strategy can be enhanced by adding a chelating agent such as ethylene diamine tetraacetic acid (EDTA) to the soap and water mix. In fact, this concept is routinely used in radiochemistry laboratories for cleaning glassware. Additionally, this strategy has a limited impact on the environment and can be deployed over a vast area.

Other strategies include the use of acetic acid (vinegar). Acetic acid is a weak organic acid that is biodegradable. Almost all cations are soluble as acetates. Vinegar has been used for years as a glass cleaner; it is effective is because some many materials are soluble in it.

Even carbonated water can be effective in complexing uranium isotopes. It turns out that uranium forms a very strong complex with the carbonate ion (this is the fizz in soft drinks). Therefore, if uranium isotopes are used in a dirty bomb, a simple application of baking soda and vinegar could prove useful.

As mentioned earlier, a graded approach should always be used (going from the simplest and cheapest to the most complex and most expensive). For example, after most mild agents have been used, one may wish to resort to strong acids such as nitric acid. Almost all inorganic nitrates are soluble, and nitric acid has the ability to oxidize and thereby "mobilize" many radio-active isotopes. In fact, nitric acid is extensively used in radiochemistry labora-tories to "digest" difficult sample types. However, because most monuments are made of marble (which is a form of calcium carbonate), this aggressive technique would used only in the worst of cases.

Other types of chemical strategies include the use of organic extractants, ion-exchange materials, foams, gels, and even aerosols.

Some types of radioisotopes are volatile, such as radioiodine and polonium. This property implies that either heat or light or both have a tendency to cause these isotopes to be suspended in a gaseous or highly mobile phase that makes them difficult to "pin down." In some respects, this property causes problems. In other cases it can be used to support cleanup. For example, simple ultra-violet (UV) radiation can cause elemental iodine to sublime (go from a solid state to a gaseous state). This property has the potential be used to suspend (using UV) radioiodine and capture it on a charcoal canister or other capture canister.

In the end, the myriad of chemical processes needs to be explored prior to a radiological event to ascertain the most effective techniques for the limited set of potential isotopes expected from a radiological device.

10.14 USE OF ISOTOPE DILUTION FOR DECONTAMINATION

The first principle of radiochemistry states that "all isotopes of the same element behave chemically the same." This powerful concept leads to what is perhaps the most powerful decontamination tool that the scientist has. This is how it works—say that a sidewalk has been contaminated with radioactive cesium-137 that has become bound in the cement. Because the cesium becomes trapped in the sand (silicates) that make up the cement, other previously mentioned techniques may not be effective at removal. Isotope dilution can offer an important means of the "trapped" radioactive cesium. Stable or nonradioactive cesium is applied to the surface and allowed to penetrate the surface. Because chemical equilibrium is dynamic this affords a means for the stable (nonradioactive isotopes) to exchange with the radioactive ones. As many more stable cesium atoms exist than the radioactive cesium atoms, and because the applied cesium on the surface can be easily removed, there will then be a propensity for the radioactive cesium to be replaced and removed. It is worth noting, however, that this technique only works with radioactive isotopes that have stable isotopes. All elements with atomic numbers between 1 and 82 (excluding elements 43 and 61) have stable isotopes. All elements above 82 have no stable isotopes. Engineers and scientists should not overlook the importance of this technique.

10.15   PRIORITIES FOR DECONTAMINATION

After a radiological release, two important considerations are examined: the protection of health and preservation of the quality of food and food production. However, the spread of contamination creates a complex situation because of the complexity of the contaminated areas. Impacts on economic, agriculture, and inhabited areas are all relevant and important considerations for priorities.

Decontamination strategies should be implemented immediately after a radiological event, and they include simple measures such as removal and cover. After a radiological release, consideration and priorities will have to be established. The following are suggested priorities for an effective decontamination strategy:

- Agriculture and plant food production
- Gathering of free foods (nuts and berries)
- Fish and marine production
- Domestic animal production
- Inhabited areas
- Drinking water

The driver behind this strategy is the potential for radioactive isotopes entering and "traveling" up the food chain. Drinking water is at the bottom because it can easily be "flushed" or discarded over a time frame that allows for minimal uptake by humans and animals. Furthermore, decision makers may have to restrict the movement, supply, or sale of certain foods or food products from within a contaminated area. The size of the area affected by food restrictions will vary on how the radiological contaminant has spread. What this implies, therefore, is that there will need to be a significant number of rapid analyses carried out by qualified laboratories. The problem with this concept is that not enough qualified radiochemistry laboratories exist in the United States to perform all the analyses that will be needed *when* a nuclear terrorist attack occurs.

CHAPTER 11

CONCLUSIONS

The greatest danger of another catastrophic attack in the United States will materialize if the world's most dangerous terrorists acquire the world's most dangerous weapons.

—The 9/11 Commission Report

11.1 NUCLEAR TERROR: ARE WE PREPARED INTERNATIONALLY?

In their report on *The World at Risk* to the White House and Congress, the Commission on the Prevention of Weapons of Mass Destruction Proliferation and Terrorism wrote the following:

The Commission believes that unless the world community acts decisively and with great urgency, it is more likely than not that a weapon of mass destruction will be used in a terrorist attack somewhere in the world by the end of 2013. . . . Compounding the nuclear threat even more is the proliferation of nuclear weapons capabilities to new states and the decision by several existing nuclear states to build up their arsenals. Such proliferation is a concern in its own right because it may increase the prospect of military crises that could lead to war and

Radiation Safety: Protection and Management for Homeland Security and Emergency Response. By L. A. Burchfield

catastrophic use of these weapons. As former Senator Sam Nunn testified to our Commission: "The risk of a nuclear weapon being used today is growing, not receding."

Clearly, the global threat is real, and it is obvious that the world has witnessed a new era of nuclear proliferations. This became apparent when it was revealed that Dr. A. Q. Khan (a Pakistani nuclear physicist) operated a "one-stop shop" for nuclear weapons and nuclear materials. With a diversity of clients such as North Korea and Iran, this nuclear proliferation has prompted a global nuclear crisis. Just a mere 68 years ago, the United States was the sole possessor of the "nuclear genie." Unfortunately, in the 21st century, all components are available for a price. Today, nuclear arms rivalries have intensified, especially in the Middle East and Asia. The open use of nuclear arms is a very real possibility by rogue nations and in a more frightening scenario by terrorist organizations.

The United States and Russia have been cooperating since the end of the Cold War by introducing new countermeasures for the security of nuclear materials and by helping to contain nuclear information and technology. This cooperation has had a degree of success; however, it has also cost the United States billions of dollars. The current economic crisis may play a detrimental role. Destabilization of the world economy has the potential of destabilizing nuclear countermeasures. Furthermore, according to the *World at Risk* report, recent intelligence reports have pointed out that Muslim activist groups have indeed intensified in number and geological location. For example, since 9/11, the numbers of terrorist groups that have aligned with al Qaeda have increased. These groups include al-Qaeda in Iraq, the Libyan Islamic Fighting Group, and the Algerian al-Qaeda in the Islamic Maghreb, which is formerly the Salafist Group for Preaching and Combat (GSPC). The bottom line is that these threats are indeed a threat to the entire world.

11.2 WHO IS INTERNATIONALLY RESPONSIBLE FOR NUCLEAR COUNTERMEASURES?

Clearly, the United States needs to take a strong leadership role in preventing nuclear technology and materials from falling into the wrong hands. However, the problem goes far beyond the leadership role of the United States. The reason is simple—the number of nation states that now possess nuclear weapons and/or are seeking development are increasing. Furthermore, terrorist groups are highly motivated in their pursuit of acquisition of nuclear materials and nuclear weapons. Illegal trafficking of nuclear materials and nuclear technology is a very serious concern that the United States alone cannot solve. The *World at Risk* report points out the following:

> The world must move with new urgency to halt the proliferation of nuclear weapons—and the United States must increase its global leadership efforts to stop the proliferation of nuclear weapons and safeguard nuclear material before it falls into the hands of terrorists. The new administration must move to revitalize the Nuclear Non-Proliferation Treaty (NPT). The nonproliferation regime embodied in the NPT has been eroded and the International Atomic Energy Agency's financial resources fall far short of its existing and expanding mandate. The amount of safeguarded nuclear bomb-making material has grown by a factor of 6 to 10 over the past 20 years, while the agency's safeguards budget has not kept pace and the number of IAEA inspections per facility has actually declined.

The Commission on the Prevention of Weapons of Mass Destruction Proliferation and Terrorism goes on to make the following recommendations:

> The United States should work internationally toward strengthening the nonproliferation regime, reaffirming the vision of a world free of nuclear weapons by:
>
> (1) imposing a range of penalties for NPT violations and withdrawal from the NPT that shift the burden of proof to the state under review for noncompliance;
>
> (2) ensuring access to nuclear fuel, at market prices to the extent possible, for non-nuclear states that agree not to develop sensitive fuel cycle capabilities and are in full compliance with international obligations;
>
> (3) strengthening the International Atomic Energy Agency, to include identifying the limitations to its safeguarding capabilities, and providing the agency with the resources and authorities needed to meet its current and expanding mandate;
>
> (4) promoting the further development and effective implementation of counterproliferation initiatives such as the Proliferation Security Initiative and the Global Initiative to Combat Nuclear Terrorism;
>
> (5) orchestrating consensus that there will be no new states, including Iran and North Korea, possessing uranium enrichment or plutonium reprocessing capability;
>
> (6) working in concert with others to do everything possible to promote and maintain a moratorium on nuclear testing;
>
> (7) working toward a global agreement on the definition of "appropriate" and "effective" nuclear security and accounting systems as legally obligated under United Nations Security Council Resolution 1540; and
>
> (8) discouraging, to the extent possible, the use of financial incentives in the promotion of civil nuclear power.

Many nation states believe that they have a right to possess nuclear weapons. Additionally, many of these nations also believe that their "world stature" and "negotiating abilities" will be enhanced by possessing nuclear weapons. In many ways this is true. One need look no further than North Korea and Iran. The key question we must all face, however, is a Will such nations be responsible in their handling of "nuclear fire" or will such materials find their way into the hands of the terrorist? Perhaps Albert Einstein said it best:

> Here, then, is the problem which we present to you, stark and dreadful and inescapable: Shall we put an end to the human race; or shall mankind renounce war?

11.3 NUCLEAR TERROR: ARE WE PREPARED NATIONALLY?

In June 2008, the U.S. Government Accountability Office (GAO) released a report concerning nuclear security, which was issued on behalf of the Committee on Homeland Security and Government Affairs and the U.S. Senate. In it, concerns were raised that terrorists could use radioactive materials and/or sealed radioactive sources to build a dirty bomb. This report was a follow-up to one issued in 2003, in which the GAO found weaknesses in the Nuclear Regulatory Commission's (NRC's) radioactive material licensing process and made recommendations for improvements.

In this latest report, the GAO assesses (1) the progress that the NRC has made in implementing the 2003 recommendations, (2) other steps the NRC has taken to improve its ability to track radioactive materials, (3) Customs and Border Protection's (CBP's) ability to detect radioactive materials at land ports of entry, and (4) CBP's ability to verify that such materials are appropriately licensed prior to entering the United States.

The GAO found that the NRC has implemented three of the six 2003 recommendations concerning security of radioactive sources. The NRC has collaborated with 35 "agreement states" (those that implement and direct radioactive source licensing and management at the state, rather than at the federal, level) to identify materials and sources in order to (1) recognize sealed sources of greatest concern, (2) enhance requirements to secure radioactive sources, and (3) ensure that security requirements are implemented.

In contrast, the NRC has made limited progress toward implementing recommendations to (1) modify its process for issuing licenses to ensure that radioactive materials cannot be purchased by those with no legitimate need, (2) determine how to effectively mitigate the potential psychological effects of malicious use of such materials, and (3) examine whether certain radioactive sources should be subject to more stringent regulations.

It is fair to say, however, that the NRC has taken four additional steps to help improve its ability to monitor and track radioactive materials. First, the NRC has created an interim national database to monitor the licensed sealed sources that contain materials that pose the greatest risk of being used in a dirty bomb. Second, the NRC is developing a National Source Tracking System to replace the interim database and provide more comprehensive, frequently updated information on potentially dangerous sources. However, this system has been delayed by 18 months and is not expected to be fully operational until January 2009. Third, the NRC is also developing a Web-based licensing system that will include more comprehensive information on all sources and materials that require NRC or state approval to possess. Finally, the NRC is developing a license verification system that will draw information from the other new systems to enable officials and vendors to verify that those seeking to bring these radioactive materials into the country or purchase them are licensed to do so.

However, these systems are more than 3 years behind schedule and may not include the licensing information, at least initially, on radioactive materials regulated by agreement states, which represent more than 80% of all U.S. licenses for such materials. The delays in the deployment and full development of these systems are especially consequential because the NRC has identified them as key to improving the control and accountability of radioactive materials.

Although the CBP has a comprehensive system in place to detect radioactive materials entering the United States at land borders, some equipment that is used to protect CBP officers is in short supply. Specifically, vehicles, cargo, and people entering the United States at most ports of entry along the Canadian and Mexican borders are scanned for radioactive materials with radiation detection equipment that can detect very small amounts of radioactive materials. However, the GAO found that personal radiation detectors are not available to all officers who need them.

Moreover, although the CBP has systems in place to verify the legitimacy of radioactive material licenses, it has not been effectively communicated to officers as to when they must contact officials to verify the license for a given sealed source. Consequently, some CBP officers are not following current guidance, and some potentially dangerous radioactive materials have entered the country without license verification.

11.4 WHAT WE KNOW ABOUT THE INEVITABLE

How will the United States or any modern nation deal with a nuclear terrorist attack? The jury is certainly still out on this frightening scenario. There are simply too many variables for anyone to predict accurately how such a nightmare would unfold. However, we do know some simple truths.

First, a even though governments around the world are tightening restriction on the handling, use, and deployment of radiological materials, it is most conceivable that naturally mined sources of radioactive materials will be "harvested" in a simple and clandestine manner, smuggled into a major metropolitan area, and unleashed. This scenario is not an "if" but a "when."

Second, how modern nations deal with such an event will require a concerted effort to educate the public to help reduce mass panic, ease fears, and decrease the tendency to overreact, especially when dealing with the inevitable cleanup and restoration that will be necessary after a nuclear terrorist attack.

Third, in this new century, nations will have to maintain a high degree of watchfulness coupled with preparedness, and followed by quick action when necessary. In the final analysis, radiation and radioactivity are an ever-present part of life—this truth is inescapable. However, mankind's fears about radiation and radioactivity have the potential to play on our psyches, if we let them.

How we cope with our fears and view our fellow man says less about who we are as individuals and more about where we are headed as a human race. Truth and fear can be viewed as opposing forces, as polarizing today as they have been in the past. The reality is that without fear, there can be no terror.

There is no fear in love; but perfect love casteth out fear: because fear hath torment. He that feareth is not made perfect in love.

—1 John 4:18 KJV

APPENDIX A

RADIOACTIVE CONTAMINATION MONITORING

Resource: Practical Radiation Technical Manual for Workplace Monitoring For Radiation and Contamination—IAEA-PRTM-1 (Rev. 1)

A radiological event [Radiological dispersion device (RDD), radiation-emitting device (RED), or improvised nuclear device (IND)] can occur at a moment's notice. First responders will be the first on the scene and the first to receive elevated radiation doses. Adequate radiation protection measures are essential for managing risks to public servants (first responders) and the general public, and these measures will be critical for saving lives.

Because of the importance of radiation protection during a nuclear terrorist attack, the concepts of radiation exposure and dose play a prominent role in the health and safety of those involved in such a disaster.

The *Planning Guidance for Protection and Recovery Following Radiological Dispersion (RDD) and Improvised Nuclear Device (IND) Incidents* was published by Homeland Security in August 2008. This guidance recommends that emergency workers receive a total effective dose of no more than 5 rem (0.05 Sv) for all reasonable actions, 10 rem (0.10 Sv) to protect valuable property necessary for public welfare (e.g., a power plant), and 25 rem (0.25 Sv) for life-saving or protection of large populations (it is unlikely that emergency workers will receive this high a level from a RDD; however, it

Radiation Safety: Protection and Management for Homeland Security and Emergency Response. By L. A. Burchfield
Copyright © 2009 John Wiley & Sons, Inc.

is conceivable that such high doses would occur from an IND). It is therefore imperative that all responders have adequate radiological monitoring equipment and know how to use it. Exposed emergency workers need to have a fundamental awareness and understanding of the risks posed by exposure to radiation and the measures for managing these risks.

A.1 INTRODUCTION

Human senses cannot detect ionizing radiation. However, excess and long-term exposure may cause adverse health effects. Hand-held radiation measuring instruments are the tools used as a first line of defense in the detection of the presence of such radiations and are often used to avoid unwarranted exposure to radiation. Using the right type of radiation detection equipment provides an effective means of limiting exposures and assists in minimizing doses.

This appendix explains the basic terminology associated with such measuring instruments and describes the principal types and respective applications to a radiological event.

If subjected to gamma radiation, different materials will in general absorb different amounts of energy. Because both physical and chemical changes can occur as a result of this absorbed radiation, the absorbed energy most often described as energy per unit mass. This then is referred to as absorbed dose or simply dose.

A fundamental distinction exists between radiation or radioactivity and dose. In general, radioactivity is measured in counts per minute (which when a correcting factor called efficiency is applied) and can be converted to disintegrations per minute. In general, the higher the activity, the higher the absorbed dose. However, it is not a one to one relationship. In fact, the absorbed dose will be a reasonable measure of the chemical or physical effects created by absorbed energy of a radioactive source. Again, the radiation source is measured in counts per unit time (usually counts per minute), and the absorbed dose is a measure of a specific amount of energy absorbed by the human body [usually measured in roentgen equivalent man (rem) or Sievert (Sv)]. In short, some types of detectors count radiation events, whereas others measure the dose to a human.

It is vital that correct radiation monitoring is carried out when there is likelihood for radiation exposure. It is equally important that the correct monitoring instrument is selected and used in an emergency setting. Competent user training is also essential for correct interpretations on the results obtained by the instrument and for assessing appropriate doses received by humans.

This appendix will be of greatest benefit when it is used to supplement a rigorous and comprehensive training program. Instrument tests and calibrations described in this appendix require the services of a qualified expert.

A.2 TYPES OF NUCLEAR DETECTION EQUIPMENT

Nuclear detection instruments are necessary to detect and quantify two fundamental types of radiation exposure: ionizing radiation sources outside the
human body, and ionizing radiation sources in a form that has the capability
of entering the human body (primarily as surface contamination such as radioactive dust, aerosols or liquids).

Four basic types of nuclear detection instruments are recommended for use
during a radiological emergency, as follows:

1. Dosimeters for measuring the cumulative external exposure
2. Aerosol or gas contamination monitors, which indicate the potential
   internal exposure when a radioactive substance is distributed within an
   atmosphere
3. Nuclear rate meter for measuring surface contamination, which indicates
   the potential internal exposure when a radioactive substance is distributed over a surface
4. Dose rate meters for measuring an immediate external human exposure
   to radiation (see Fig. A.1)

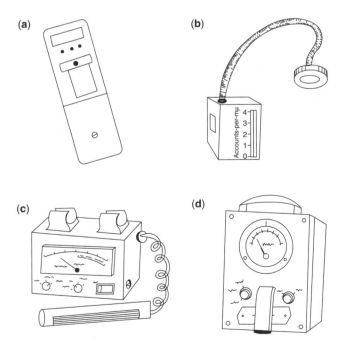

Figure A.1. Radiation monitoring instruments include: (a) Dosimeters. (b) Airborne contamination meters and gas monitors. (c) Surface contamination meters. (d) Dose rate meters.

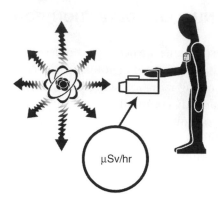

Figure A.2. A dose rate meter measures external hazards in units of dose equivalent rate. Dose rate meters provide direct measurements of external exposure.

A.3 DOSE RATE METERS

A dose rate meter measures absorbed energy from penetrating radiation. A suitable and efficient instrument that is matched to the specific task should be capable of providing direct readings of the dose equivalent rate in microsieverts per hour (μSv/hr or mSv/hr). A smaller number of instruments indicate the absorbed dose rate in micrograys per hour (mGy/hr). These instruments usually respond only to X-rays, gamma, and/or beta radiations. Specialized instruments are necessary to measure neutron dose equivalent rates. Older units of dose rate—millirem per hour (mrem/hr), millirad per hour (mrad/hr), and milliroentgen per hour (mR/hr)—are still displayed on some instruments (10 mSv/hr is equivalent to 1 mrem/hr).

Dose rate meters may not be able to provide an accurate response to rapidly changing or pulsed radiation fields. Integrating dose rate meters and dosimeters are more appropriate in such circumstances (see Fig. A.2).

A.4 DOSIMETERS

Dosimeters measure the total energy absorbed as a consequence of exposure to ionizing radiation. Several types of dosimeters are available, including thermoluminescent dosimeters (TLDs), optically stimulated luminescence (OSL), electronic dosimeter, film dosimeter, and direct ion storage. TLDs store radiation energy in a crystal such as lithium fluoride that is later "read" by heating the crystal and measuring the glow of light that is proportional to the radiation level that first struck the crystal.

OSLs are a relatively new technology that differs from TLDs in that trapped charges are released using optical rather than thermal energy.

Electronic dosimeters measure radiation exposure on a real-time basis and provide immediate dose rate readings. Depending on the environment, parameters can be set on the device to warn individuals that they are approaching a certain limit of exposure.

Film dosimeters are processed in the same way as photographic film. A calibrated light source and sensitive detectors are used to measure the amount of light that can pass through the film. This information determines the quantity and type of radiation exposing the film.

Direct ion storage measures radiation by absorbing charges into a miniature (MOSFET) ion chamber. The dosimeter can be instantaneously processed and read by an on-site reader.

Personnel dosimeters should be worn by all emergency responders while in a radiological zone to assess their radiation exposure. Passive dosimeters routinely monitor cumulative doses that result from an external exposure. Active dosimeters provide an immediate reading of the dose in microsieverts (μSv) and may also provide an immediate alarm signal when the measured dose approaches a value preset by the manufacturer or the health physics specialist.

Integrating dose rate meters and dosimeters can be used to assess an external exposure which is rapidly changing, for example: (1) a task of short duration has to be carried out in the presence of high dose rates, and (2) the source [e.g., high dose rates while near the release point of a radiological dispersion device (RDD)] emits radiation within a short distance of a radiological device (Fig. A.3).

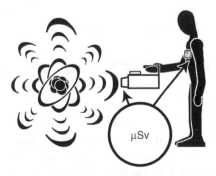

Figure A.3. Personnel dosimeters and integrating dose rate meters have the ability to measure the dose equivalent caused by an external hazard that is rapidly changing. Dosimeters, however, provide a measurement of cumulative exposure to radiation.

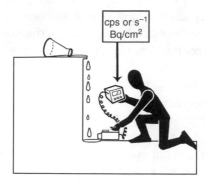

Figure A.4. Surface contamination meters are used to detect and measure radioactive substances on surfaces. A surface contamination meter can indicate a potential for uptake and internal exposure to radiation.

A.5 SURFACE CONTAMINATION METERS

Surface contamination meters are used to detect the presence of radioactive substances on accessible surfaces. Even low concentrations of such substances may present a potential internal exposure. However, each instrument will have detection efficiencies that range from near 0% to 30% (at best) depending on what types of radionuclides are present. For example, alpha-emitting radionuclides present the most significant challenge in being measured because almost anything stops an alpha.

Measurements must be made using a calibrated instrument with the best available, predetermined detection efficiency for the contaminant. The measurements, in counts per second (cps or s^{-1}), need to be converted to becquerels per square centimeter (Bq/cm^2).

Some surface contamination meters are programmable. The user sets the instrument's likely response to the radionuclide in use and obtains a direct measurement of surface contamination (in Bq/cm^2) (Fig. A.4).

A.6 AIRBORNE CONTAMINATION METERS AND GAS MONITORS

Airborne contamination meters are used to detect radioactive aerosols that may be present after a nuclear detonation or a chemical explosion involving a RDD. These may be dispersion aerosols (dusts), condensation aerosols (smoke), or liquid aerosols (mists). Fallout particles from a nuclear weapons detonation or improvised nuclear device (IND) liberate large particles from 50 to 200 μm (1/1000th of a millimeter). This means that fallout from nuclear weapons or INDs can be easily filtered and/or blocked from entering a shelter or well-sealed house. Particles from an RDD can be on the submicron level, which means that Hepa filters must be used to remove them from contaminated air. Submicron particles also present a mechanism for easily entering the lungs. Thus, although an RDD presents a much smaller activity level than an IND or nuclear detonation, the harm on a very localized scale can be more severe to those who breathe these much smaller particles.

Instruments for monitoring airborne contamination normally draw suspect contaminated air at a constant rate through a filter or past a detector with instantaneous feedback. The problem with the former is that filters need to be measured elsewhere. The advantage to air filters is that they can be retained for additional analyses.

Gas monitoring detectors provide monitoring by simply moving the radioactive gas past a detector. The advantage of gas monitors is that they give direct and immediate feedback of the presence of airborne radioactive gases. In general, most gas monitoring systems measure in units of becquerels per cubic meter (Bq/m^3). Airborne contamination meters and gas monitors may be used to assess airborne contamination in the event of a radiological event. More than likely, such instruments will be flown on small aircraft.

It is highly recommended that emergency response personnel use a personal breathing apparatus while in a declared "hot zone" after a radiological event. However, if such equipment is not available or is not used, one may wish to use personnel air samplers (PAS). A PAS is simply a small pump usually worn on a belt that pulls air through a filter at chest level. PAS systems are used to monitor the more significant hazard within the breathing zone of an individual worker. These instruments are often passive devices that do not provide immediate measurements. They only provide a total measurement of radioactivity that is trapped on a filter; these results may not necessarily reflect actual intake by the emergency response personnel.

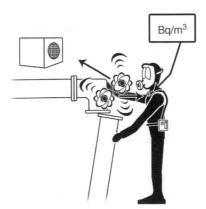

Figure A.5. Personnel and static samplers as well as gas monitors are used to monitor airborne contamination. Airborne contamination meters are used to detect and measure particulate radioactivity in the atmosphere. Gas monitors are used to detect and measure radioactive gases in the atmosphere.

Some instruments can detect the radionuclides in real time and provide an alarm signal when the radioactivity reaches a preset level (Fig. A.5).

A.7   BASIC RADIATION INSTRUMENT COMPONENTS

Commercially available radiation detection instruments are often described and procured on the basis of their essential components. The key components are as follows:

The Detector. The detector contains a medium that absorbs radiation energy and converts it into a signal. Electrical charge usually forms the signal. Common detectors include the following:

- Gas filled detectors
- Ionization chambers
- Proportional counters
- Geiger-Müller counters
- Scintillation counters
- Solid-state detectors

The Amplifier. The signals from a detector may need to be electronically boosted or amplified.

The Processor. According to the type of instrument, the processor may be a device to measure the size or number of signals produced by the detector. It may also translate the quantity measured into appropriate radiological units.

The Display. The measurement is presented either in a digital format or as an analog display showing a pointer on a graduated scale.

The Radiation. Ionizing radiations (alpha or beta particles, gamma rays, X-rays, or neutrons) that enter the detector need to be absorbed to be detected.

The Ionization. The process in which the detector medium absorbs radiation energy.

A.8   IONIZATION CHAMBERS AS GAS-FILLED DETECTORS

Ionization chambers, like proportional counters and Geiger-Müller counters, are gas-filled detectors. The essential components of these detectors are as follows:

A—a container or detector wall that encloses the gas. The material used strongly influences the instrument's performance and use.

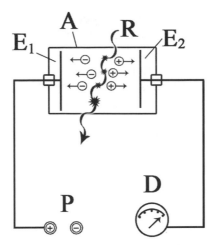

Figure A.6. Principal components of an ionization chamber. Ionization chambers, proportional counters, and Geiger-Müller counters are gas-filled detectors operating on the fact that radiation causes ionization in the gas filling.

$E_{1,2}$—electrodes (a positive anode and a negative cathode) physically separated and across which a fixed potential difference (voltage) is maintained.

P—powers supply (battery).

D—a display.

Ionization counters can operate with different gas fillings and gas pressures; however, sometimes air is used at atmospheric pressure and temperature. The amount of energy from radiation that a gas absorbs is proportional to the number of ions generated within the gas. These ions migrate to an oppositely charged particle and create a flow of electrical current. The shape and duration of the electrical pulse determines how much activity and what type of radiation has entered the detection chamber (short duration pulses are usually counted as alpha particles, and long pulses are counted as beta particles) (Fig. A.6).

A.9 PROPORTIONAL COUNTERS AND GAS AMPLIFICATION

Gas proportional counters normally include a mixture of inert and organic gases. However, other gases may be used to form special detectors. For example, incorporating boron trifluoride (BF_3) permits the detection of neutrons. Boron has a high nuclear cross section for the absorption of neutrons. When a neutron is absorbed, it causes the BF_3 to be ionized (with most gases neutrons have little if any interactions).

Gas proportional detectors can be operated at elevated gas pressures to provide higher detection efficiencies for X-rays, gamma rays, and beta radiations. The high voltages applied also increase their sensitivity to low dose rates. One new type of gamma detector uses high-pressure xenon gas.

Higher voltages cause the ions, which are created by ionizing radiations, to accelerate as they approach the electrodes. The fast moving negative ions in turn cause secondary and tertiary ionization events. This principle is gas amplification. The number of ions collected by the electrode will be proportional to the number produced by the radiation, hence the term proportional counter. The detector's output is a pulse of charge when the ions are collected on the electrode.

Gas amplification occurs in both proportional and Geiger-Müller counters. Proportional counters and Geiger-Müller counters use gas amplification to increase the sensitivity of the detector.

A.10 GEIGER-MÜLLER COUNTERS AND DETECTOR OUTPUT

Geiger-Müller counters (also called GM or sometimes Geigers) contain a low-pressure inert gas and traces of an organic or halogen gas referred to as the quenching agent. The quenching agent is necessary because it helps to "quench" the cascade events within secondary and tertiary ionizations. It the detector did not have quenching agents, the detector would become "swamped" and would not recover easily. These multiple ionizations would cause continual electrical discharge within the detector.

The significant difference among a GM's electrodes is high and sufficient to cause an almost complete ionization of the detector gas from a single primary ionization. A brief reduction of the voltage then allows the detector's recovery.

The graph illustrates the relative response of gas-filled detectors to a single ionizing particle. The number of ions collected (n) is plotted against the detector voltage (V). The detector regions are indicated.

A—ionization chambers. Above a minimum voltage, the few primary ions do not recombine and are collected.

B—proportional counters. The detector's response increases with increasing ionization.

C—Geiger-Müller counters. The avalanche of ions collected is independent of the primary ionization.

A GM's output differs from that of other gas-filled detectors. Pulses of electrical charge result as a count rate that is proportional to the radiation fluence

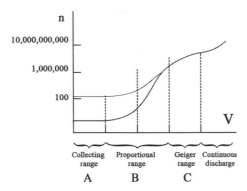

Figure A.7. Typical output of gas-filled detectors in response to single primary ionizations from different types of radiation events. Gas-filled detectors need to operate at the appropriate voltages to function properly.

(or intensity of particles) and does not determine the energy of the radiation. Many types of GM detectors provide an audio output in the form of "clicks" or "chirps." Gas-filled detectors need to operate at proper voltages to operate properly (Fig. A.7).

A.11   PRACTICAL IONIZATION CHAMBER INSTRUMENTS

Ionization chambers are used to manufacture accurate dose rate meters as well as integrating dose rate meters. A typical construction is illustrated, as follows:

A—the cylindrical detector wall serves as the cathode (negative electrode) and is normally made of air-equivalent, carbon-coated plastic or aluminum.

B—the axial anode (positive electrode).

C—beta window made of thin foil ($3-7 \, \text{mg/cm}^2$).

D—protective buildup cap ($200-300 \, \text{mg/cm}^3$) made of toughened plastic or aluminum.

The buildup cap is used to improve the detection efficiency when measuring high-energy photon radiations. It is removed when measuring dose rates caused by low energy photons (10 to 100 keV) and beta radiations.

Detector volumes of a few hundred cubic centimeters are needed to measure exposures in nanocoulombs per hour (nC/hr). The processor converts these units to the appropriate radiation dose rates from about $10 \, \mu\text{Sv/hr}$. Ambient variations of temperature, humidity, and air pressure will affect the detector and should be corrected as appropriate. Care should also be exercised in the

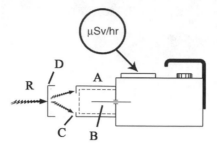

Figure A.8. Ionization chambers provide an accurate measurement of dose rate.

use of radio-emitting devices because in some instances detectors may be interfered with by radio signals (Fig. A.8).

A.12   PRACTICAL PROPORTIONAL COUNTERS

Portable dose and dose rate meters that incorporate proportional counters are not common. Some proportional counters can measure low dose rates. In most cases, they are smaller than equivalent ionization chambers; however, proportional counters need a highly stable power, and continuous gas flow makes their use as a field instrument not practical. Proportional counter's enhanced sensitivity is best used for measuring surface contamination. Meters are available that may contain detectors as large as $1500\,\text{cm}^2$.

Compared with Geiger counters, proportional counters have a better response to low-energy photons and a higher sensitivity to beta particles.

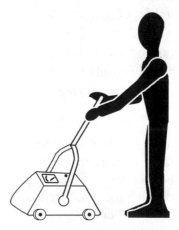

Figure A.9. A large-area proportional counter incorporated in a "sidewalk" contamination meter. Proportional counters are used to measure dose rate, airborne radioactivity, and surface contamination.

However, Geiger instruments are less costly for measuring dose rates from penetrating radiation.

Proportional counters are mostly used in the laboratory. The detector's applications include spectrometry (Frisch grid detectors), neutron detection, discrimination between ionizing particles (e.g., alpha and beta), and absolute measurements of the activity by applying an appropriate efficiency (Fig. A.9).

A.13   PRACTICAL GEIGER-MÜLLER COUNTERS

Geiger-Müller counters are manufactured in a range of shapes, sizes, sensitivities, and detection geometries. The detector requires only a moderately stable voltage, a simple amplifier, and other inexpensive components, which include a rate meter, to construct a useful instrument. Common forms include the following:

The Geiger tube. A cylindrical tube (often of glass about 30 mg/cm^2 thick) surrounded with a tubular cathode and an axial wire anode. As a side window detector, the tube is enclosed within a metal shield that has a shutter. The shield protects the tube and provides a means to discriminate between penetrating and nonpenetrating radiations.

The end window Geiger tube. A cylindrical thin metal body forms the cathode which is sealed at one end by a thin window of about 2 mg/cm^2. Alpha, beta, and photon radiations can be detected through the window; however, alphas have poor detection efficiencies.

GM counters create a pulsed output that triggers an audible signal. GM counters have the ability to respond rapidly to varying dose rates. Geiger counters can suffer from "saturated" events when exceptionally high dose rates are present. In these potentially hazardous situations, these instruments become paralyzed and stop to functioning. Selected circuits (within some types of detectors) make sure that a full-scale reading is sustained under such conditions.

A.14   SCINTILLATION COUNTERS

The essential components of a scintillation counter are as follows:

S—Scintillator. A phosphor contained within a nontransparent enclosure. Ionizing radiations interact with the scintillator, which in turn immediately converts some absorbed energy into photons.

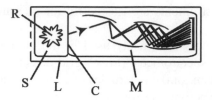

Figure A.10. Principal components of a scintillation counter. Scintillation counters contain a phosphor and a photomultiplier.

L—Light guide transfers the scintillation to the photocathode (C) of the photomultiplier tube (M).

C—Photocathode is a type of vacuum tube that is translucent, with a light-sensitive coating of material (e.g., antimony doped with cesium) on the photomultiplier window. When light is absorbed, it produces electrons that cascade down the dynodes and are multiplied by a factor of 1E6 to 1E7.

M—Photomultiplier tube includes electrodes called dynodes. A successively increased potential difference (about 2000 V overall) draws electrons to each dynode in turn. The number of electrons increases at each dynode. The number of electrons is multiplied by a factor of 1 million to 10 million.

Scintillation devices on the front side of the photomultiplier tube turn the light into electrons. They include materials such as solid organics (anthracene and stilbene), liquid scintillants, and solid plastic scintillants and activated inorganic crystals such as sodium iodide and cesium iodide, which are activated by trace amounts of thallium [NaI(Tl) and CsI(Tl)] (Fig. A.10).

A.15   PRACTICAL BULK SCINTILLATION COUNTERS

The very wide variety of phosphors in a multitude of sizes, geometries, and sensitivities can be combined with photomultiplier tubes that range from 6 to 300 mm in diameter to form a great diversity of scintillation counter instruments.

Organic and inorganic phosphors with densities close to 1000 times greater than those of gas-filled detectors are used to detect gamma and X-rays with very high sensitivities. Crystals of up to 40 cm in diameter and 40 cm in thickness exist, but crystals of a diameter between 1 cm and 7.5 cm are used regularly. For radiation that is incident perpendicular to a 2.5-cm-thick NaI(Tl) crystal, the detection efficiency is about 37% for 1 MeV photons. The efficiency rises to nearly 100% at energies below 200 keV.

For detectors of sufficient size, the scintillations will be proportional to the energy of the incident photons, which allows them to be used for low-resolution gamma spectrometry. The scintillation rate is proportional to the radiation fluence and not the dose rate. However, scintillation dose rate meters that operate over limited energy ranges, can indicate low and high dose rates even at low photon energies.

The photomultiplier's demand for a stable voltage supply and high-component costs make these instruments relatively expensive. Their bulk, weight, and vulnerability to shock also limit their usefulness. However, portable instruments are now available which provide spectrometry as well as dosimetry.

Lithium iodide activated by europium [LiI(Eu)] and silver activated zinc sulphide [ZnS(Ag)] in a boron loaded plastic scintillator are used for neutron detection.

A.16   PRACTICAL SCINTILLATION COUNTER CONTAMINATION MONITORS

Highly sensitive surface contamination detectors incorporate a wide range of phosphor arrangements. In addition to the gamma phosphors, other examples include the following: (1) zinc sulphide [ZnS(Ag)] powder coatings (5–10 mg/cm^2) on glass or plastic substrates or coated directly onto the photomultiplier window for detecting alpha and other heavy particles; (2) cesium iodide [CsI(Tl)] that is thinly machined (0.25 mm) and that may be molded into various shapes; and (3) plastic phosphors in thin sheets or powders fixed to a glass base for beta detection.

Probes and their linked rate meters tend not to be rugged. Photomultiplier tubes are sensitive to breakage and are affected by nearby magnetic fields. Even minor damage to the thin foil through which radiation enters the detector allows ambient light to enter and swamp the photomultiplier. Cables connecting rate-meters and probes are also a common problem.

Low-energy beta emitters such as tritium can be dissolved in a liquid scintillator to be detected. Liquid scintillation counter instruments can be designed to be highly sensitive to alpha and beta particles.

A.17   SOLID STATE DETECTORS

Solid-state detectors are made of semiconductor materials such as high-purity silicon and high purity germanium. Two groups of detectors are junction detectors and bulk conductivity detectors.

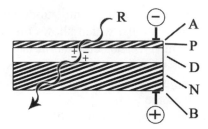

Figure A.11. Principles of surface barrier solid-state counter—shown enlarged and in section. Solid-state counters contain semiconductor devices.

Junction detectors are either the diffused junction or the surface barrier type: An impurity is either diffused into, or spontaneously oxidized onto, a prepared surface of intrinsic material to change a layer of "p-type" semiconductor from or to "n-type." When a voltage (reverse bias) is applied to the surface barrier detector, as shown, it behaves like a solid ionization chamber.

A—very thin metal (gold) electrode

P—thin layer of p-type semiconductor

D—depletion region, 3–10 mm thick formed by the voltage, is free of charge in the absence of ionizing radiations

N—n-type semiconductor

B—thin metal electrode that provides a positive potential at the n-type semiconductor

Bulk conductivity detectors are formed from intrinsic semiconductors of very high-bulk-resistivity such as CdS and CdSe. They also operate like ionization counters but with a higher density than gases and a 10-fold greater ionization per unit absorbed dose. More amplification by the detector creates outputs of about 1 μA at 10 mSv/hr (Fig. A.11).

A.18   PRACTICAL SOLID STATE DETECTORS

The main applications for semiconductor detectors are in the laboratory for the spectrometry of both heavy charged (alpha) particle and gamma radiations. However, energy compensated PIN diodes and special photodiodes are being used as pocket electronic (active) dosimeters.

Specifically combined thin and thick detectors offer the means to identify charged particles. For example, these detectors are used to check for plutonium in air, discriminating against alpha particles arising from natural radioactivity. These detectors can also be used for monitoring for radon daughter products in air. Their small physical size and insensitivity to gamma radiation have found novel applications: alpha monitoring inside nuclear fuel flasks and checking sealed radium sources for leakage.

Bulk conductivity detectors can measure high dose rates but with minute-long response times. A high purity germanium detector operates at $-170°C$ and is capable of a high resolution. The temperature dependence and high cost add to their impracticality as a field deployed instrument.

A.19 TESTING DOSE RATE METERS

Most dose rate meters are "type tested" by manufacturers and independent laboratories. The results may be found in the technical literature. In addition to the instrument's description, its directional and energy response as well as accuracy may be reported over the appropriate dose rate and energy ranges.

Each instrument must be tested before first use, at regular intervals (annually), and after any repair that may have affected the instrument's performance. These tests are conducted by qualified experts using calibrated radiation sources. The objectives are as follows:

- To insure that instruments are operating according to specifications. Other tests are needed to check for the instrument's mechanical and electrical components.
- Instrument checks must be performed to determine the absolute bias error. Errors within the $+20\%$ range may be acceptable and thus corrected; however, above this uncertainty, call the instrument's performance into question, and it should be recalibrated or replaced.
- The instrument should also be checked for linearity of response over a range that eclipses the ranges expected.

A certificate relating to the last formal test or calibration should be kept with the instrument. Furthermore, the end user should carry routine checks on the instrument. Some instruments have installed check sources, but the regular measurement of a known dose rate serves the purpose. The battery condition should be checked each time the instrument is used.

Calibrated sources and the inverse square law are applied to the testing of dose rate meters. Dose rate meters must be formally tested and calibrated at appropriate intervals.

A.20 PROCEDURES FOR USING A DOSE RATE METER

Before attempting to make a radiation measurement, it is important for the user to be entirely familiar with the features and controls of the instrument. The following instructions are recommended for the first responder and/or radiological technician:

Verify performance

- Check the test or calibration certificate. Confirm that the last formal test date, test conditions, and result are satisfactory. Check the last routine test result.
- Assess the radiation to be measured. Judge whether the instrument is suitable to obtain the measurement required.
- Set the instrument's parameters. Test the battery, adjust the detector voltage, and set the zero as necessary.

Obtain the measurement

- On multirange instruments, start on the maximum and then switch successively to lower ranges until an appropriate reading is obtained.
- Check the range setting and note the reading.
- Repeat the measurement with and without a buildup cap or with a beta/gamma shutter open and closed.
- Check the stability of the readings for different orientations of the instrument.

Assess the result

Decide whether any factors have influenced the result, such as follows:

- A nonisotropic or pulsing radiation field
- Temperature, humidity, or air-pressure effects
- Interference from radiofrequency or magnetic fields

Apply correction factors

- Multiply the reading by any relevant correction or calibration factors.

Record the result

- Decide whether the result is reasonable by comparison with previous measurements or calculations.
- Keep a written record of the conclusions.

It is important to understand the controls and the display of a dose rate meter before attempting to use it. The user of a dose rate meter must understand the instrument used and follow a procedure to obtain a meaningful measurement.

A.21 TESTING AND CALIBRATION OF SURFACE CONTAMINATION METERS

Each type of surface contamination meter is designed to measure a specific range of contaminants. Its response to contamination will depend on the following:

- The type and energy of the radiation. Each radionuclide has (in general) a unique signature of decay energies and half-life.
- The instrument's absolute counting efficiency, which is determined by the window area and thickness as well as the dimensions of any protective screen.
- The detection geometry, which includes the surface area of the detector, the type of surface contaminated, and the air gap between the surface and the detector.
- Instrument electrical noise and ageing of the instrument's components.

Instrument checks should be performed before the first use. Calibrations should be performed annually and after any repair that may have affected the instrument's performance. Calibrations should be conducted by qualified experts using calibration sources with an active area similar in dimensions to the detector. The radionuclide used should have similar decay mode and energy characteristics as the potential contaminants.

It is a good practice to keep the calibration data with the instrument. Check sources are generally attached to the case of the instrument to provide a "ready-made" check source. The battery condition should be checked each time the instrument is used.

A surface contamination meter is tested against a calibrated source. Surface contamination meters must be formally tested and calibrated at appropriate intervals.

A.22 USE OF A SURFACE CONTAMINATION METER

A suitable surface contamination meter should be available wherever unsealed radioactive substances such as liquids and powders may be present.

Caution is taken to avoid contact of the instrument with potentially contaminated surfaces.

Instruments that have a detachable probe provide versatility in decay mode detection (alpha, beta, and gamma). Flat surfaces (bench tops, floors, etc.) that are easily accessible are routinely monitored with surface contamination meters. Liquids or thick surfaces (tiles, carpet, flooring, etc.) will cause sever attenuation of alpha and beta particles and low-energy gamma emitters. An understanding of the magnitude of attenuation will be important to determine activity levels properly.

The user of a surface contamination meter must understand the instrument used and follow a procedure to obtain a meaningful measurement.

A.23 PROCEDURES FOR USING A SURFACE CONTAMINATION METER

Verify   Verify that the test or calibration certificate is valid (within less than a year since calibration). Confirm that the last formal test date, test conditions, and result are satisfactory. Perform an instrument check.

Determine Instrument Selection   Determine that the selected instrument is suitable for the potential radioactive contaminant.

Set Instrument Parameters   Set the instrument's parameters. Test the battery, adjust the detector voltage, and set the zero as necessary. Place the instrument setting on the minimum setting and graduate to a higher setting as needed.

Measure Background   Measure the background count rate (in counts per second) at a distance that is more than 1 m from the contaminated surface.

Measure the Contaminated Surface   Measure the contaminated surface moving the detector at a speed appropriate to the detector's capabilities. It is important to scan the instrument over the surface at a distance that avoids contact (generally 0.5 cm or approximately 1/4 in).

Convert from Counts to Disintegration   The net counts are calculated by subtracting the measured background. Next, an appropriate efficiency correction is applied to convert cps to dps (a typical efficiency correction will be 0.02 to 0.3 with units of dps/cps). The data is corrected by an appropriate attenuation correction (attenuation factors correct for the blocking of the incident radiation between the source and the detector; factors range from 1.0 to .05 and thereby should be divided into the net count rate). Lastly, the appropriate correction factor is applied to convert total activity (Bq or dps) to a value of surface contamination (in Bq/cm^2).

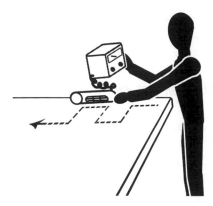

Figure A.12. Working surfaces are surveyed to detect potential surface contamination. Surface contamination meters must be suitable for detecting the contaminant to determine the potential internal exposure in the workplace.

Assess the Result   Determine whether any factors could influence the result, such as the curvature of the surface that should be applied. Review the results and assure that they are reasonable.

Record the result   Compare the result with expectations or previous measurements. Keep a written record of the conclusions (Fig. A.12).

A.24 SPECIAL SURFACE CONTAMINATION MONITORING TECHNIQUES

Two categories of surface contamination are as follows: fixed and removable. Removable is the activity that can be removed via a smear or swipe sample and that which can be removed by decontamination. Activity that cannot be removed is labeled as "fixed."

Surface contamination meters indicate the total contamination, which includes that which is fixed to the surface and that which is removable. Total contamination may constitute an external radiation dose hazard; however, that which is removable presents a potential for an internal radiation dose hazard vis-à-vis inhalation. The direct measurement may suffice as an indicator of the potential for an overall hazard; however, multiple measurements must be made to assess fixed and removable.

The removable contamination may be assessed by using a moistened filter paper to wipe an area of contaminated surface and by measuring the amount of activity on the wipe. It is normally assumed that only about 10% of the removable contamination transfers to the smear. The measured activity is multiplied by 10 and divided by the area wiped to complete the assessment.

In situations where surface access is limited or where surfaces are contaminated by alpha or low-energy beta emitters, smears are generally counted in a liquid scintillation counter.

A.25 THE MEASUREMENT OF AIRBORNE CONTAMINATION

Airborne contamination meters may be grouped as follows:

- PASs that draw 2–4 L/min of air through a filter; battery-powered samplers that sample about 10 L/min; generator-powered samplers that typically operate at 30, 60, or 100 L/min.
- "High-volume" samplers that can sample 1000 L/min for environmental rather than workplace monitoring.

Passive air samplers may readily demonstrate the presence of aerosols in the immediate vicinity, but the interpretation of the results is very difficult. Static samplers are influenced by the proximity of building surfaces, and PAS filters risk contact and being wiped or contaminated. Filter papers must also be handled with care before and after sampling to ensure that they are kept flat, undamaged, and not contaminated by contact. Additionally, filters should be preweighed and postweighed to determine attenuation factors from buildup of smoke, dust, and so on. By marking the potentially active face of the filter prior to use, better care may be provided during the filter's transfer to a laboratory for the activity to be measured. Notes should be taken of the sampling period, the flow rates at the start and finish, and sampling location(s).

If the contaminant is identified, air sampling may determine the total airborne activity concentration (in Bq/m^3). The assessment will include respirable and nonrespirable aerosols. To assess the actual risk to an exposed worker, an analysis of the particle size or a respirable particle collector is required.

A portable, generator-powered static air sampler can be used to sample particles. Airborne contamination measurements depend on an appropriate choice of sampler and the careful handling of filters.

A.26 CRITERIA FOR THE SELECTION OF MONITORING INSTRUMENTS

Factors that influence the choice of radiation monitoring instruments for any particular application include the following:

- Radiation type to be measured
- Dose, dose rate, or contamination measurements

- Energy response of the instrument
- Unwanted responses and overload performance
- Sensitivity and range of measurements required
- Instrument response speed
- Logarithmic/linear analog scales or digital displays and ease of use
- Illumination settings and/or audible output
- Cautionary indicators for response in ambient temperatures, humidity, radiofrequencies, magnetic fields, and so on
- Intrinsic safety in explosive/flammable locations
- Ease of decontamination
- Battery availability and life expectancy
- Size, weight, and portability
- Ruggedness, reliability, and serviceability
- Initial and ongoing maintenance costs

Wide ranges of radiation-monitoring instruments are manufactured. The instrument used to monitor the workplaces must be appropriate and efficient for the application.

LIST OF ACRONYMS AND ABBREVIATIONS

A	Atomic mass number
AFB	Air Force Base
AFRRI	Armed Forces Radiobiology Research Institute
ALARA	As low as reasonably achievable—A process to control or manage radiation exposure to individuals as well as the release of radioactive material to the environment so that doses are as low as social, technical, economic, practical, and public welfare considerations permit.
ALI	Annual limit of intake
AMS	Aerial Measuring System—A Department of Energy (DOE) technical asset that consists of both fixed wing and helicopter systems for measuring radiation on the ground; a deployable asset of the Nanoscale Interdisciplinary Research Team (NIRT).
ANL	Argonne National Laboratory
ANSI	American National Standards Institute
Anti-C	Anti-contamination clothing
ARG	Accident Response Group
ARM	Area radiation monitor

ARS	Acute radiation syndrome
ATN	Acute tubular necrosis
BAT	Biodosimetry Assessment Tool
BNL	Brookhaven National Laboratory
Bq	Bequerels—1 Bq = 1 disintegration per second
BWR	Boiling water reactor
CAM	Continuous air monitor
CDC	Center for Disease Control
CDE	Committed dose equivalent
CEDE	Committed effective dose equivalent
CERCLA	Comprehensive Environmental Response, Compensation, and Liability Act, commonly known as Superfund. This legislation was enacted by Congress in 1980 to protect households and communities from abandoned toxic waste sites.
CFR	Code of Federal Regulations
Ci	Curie—a unit of measure of radioactivity—1 Ci = 3.7E10 dps or Bq
CMHT	Consequence Management Home Team
CMO	Consequence Management Official
CMRT	Consequence Management Response Team
CMS	Consequence Management Site Restoration, Cleanup, and Decontamination Subgroup
CNS	Central nervous system
CPM	Counts per minute
Cs	Cesium
CV	Cardiovascular
DEST	Domestic Emergency Support Team—A technical advisory team designed to predeploy and assist the Federal Bureau of Investigation (FBI) Special Agent in Charge. The DEST may deploy after an incident to assist the FBI.
DFO	Disaster field office
DHS	U.S. Department of Homeland Security
DIL	Derived intervention level—The concentration of a radionuclide in food expressed in Becquerel/kg that, if present throughout the relevant period of time (with no intervention), could lead to an individual receiving a radiation dose equal to the protective action guide (PAG).
DNA	Deoxyribonucleic acid
DOC	U.S. Department of Commerce
DOD	U.S. Department of Defense
DOE	U.S. Department of Energy

DOE/HQ	DOE Headquarters
DOI	U.S. Department of Interior
DOJ	U.S. Department of Justice
DOS	U.S. Department of State
DOT	U.S. Department of Transportation
dpm	Disintegrations per minute
DRD	Direct reading dosimeter
DRL	Derived response level—A level of radioactivity in an environmental medium that would be expected to produce a dose equal to its corresponding PAG.
DTPA	Diethylenetriaminepentaacetate
ECN	Emergency communications network
EDE	Effective dose equivalent
EICC	Emergency Information and Coordination Center
EMP	Electromagnetic pulse—Electromagnetic radiation from a nuclear explosion.
EMS	Emergency medical service
EO	Executive order
EOC	Emergency operations center—A response entity's central command and control center for carrying out emergency management functions.
EOF	Emergency operations facility
EOP	Emergency operating procedure
EPA	U.S. Environmental Protection Agency
EPR	Emergency preparedness and response
EPZ	Environmental protection zone
ERDO	Emergency Response Duty Officer
ERDS	Emergency Response Database System
ERT	Emergency Response Team
ERT-A	Emergency Response Team—Advance Element
ESF	Emergency support function—The ESFs provide the structure for coordinating federal interagency support for domestic incident response.
FBI	Federal Bureau of Investigation, U.S. Department of Justice.
FCO	Federal Coordinating Officer—Appointed by the Director of the Federal Emergency Management Agency, on behalf of the President, to coordinate federal assistance to a state affected by a disaster or emergency.
FDA	Food and Drug Administration, U.S. Department of Health and Human Services.
FECC	Federal Emergency Communications Coordinator

FEMA	Federal Emergency Management Agency
FISH	Florescence in situ hybridization
FRERP	Federal Radiological Emergency Response Plan
FRMAC	Federal Radiological Monitoring and Assessment Center— A coordinating center for federal, state, and local field personnel performing radiological monitoring and assessment—specifically, providing data collection, data analysis and interpretation, and finished products to decision makers. The FRMAC is a deployable asset of the NIRT administered by the DOE. For more information, see http://www.nv.doe.gov/nationalsecurity/homelandsecurity/frmac/default.htm.
FRMAP	Federal Radiological Monitoring and Assessment Plan
FRN	Federal Register Notice
FRP	Federal Response Plan
FRPCC	Federal Radiological Preparedness Coordinating Committee
G-CSF	Granulocyte colony-stimulating factor
GeLi	Lithium drifted germanium—a type of gamma spectrometer that is now obsolete.
GFPC	Gas flow proportional counter
GI	Gastrointestinal
GIS	Geographical information systems
GM-CSF	Granulocyte-macrophage colony-stimulating factor
GPS	Global positioning system
GSA	General Services Administration
GVHD	Graft-versus-host disease
Gy	One gray is equal to an absorbed dose (mean energy imparted to a unit of matter mass) of 1 J/kg. 1 gray (Gy) = 10,000 erg/g = 100 rad.
HAZMAT	Hazardous material
HAZWOPER	Hazardous Waste Operations and Emergency Response Standard (29 CFR 1910.120)
HHS	U.S. Department of Health and Human Services
HLW	High-level waste
HP	Health physicist
HPGe	High-purity germanium—This refers to a specific type of gamma spectrometer.
HSPD	Homeland Security Presidential Directive—Executive order issued to the federal agencies by the President on matters pertaining to homeland security.
HUD	Department of Housing and Urban Development

I	Iodine
IAEA	International Atomic Energy Agency
IATA	International Air Transport Association
IC/US	Incident Command/Unified Command—A system to integrate various necessary functions to respond to emergencies. The system is widely used by local responders. Under Unified Command, multiple jurisdictional authorities are integrated.
ICP	Incident Command Post—The field location where the primary functions are performed. The ICP may be colocated with the incident base or other incident facilities.
ICPMS	Inductively coupled plasma mass spectrometer
ICRP	International Commission on Radiological Protection
ICS	Incident Command System—A standardized, on-scene, all-hazard incident management concept. ICS is based on a flexible, scalable response organization providing a common framework within which people can work together effectively.
IND	Improvised nuclear device—An illicit nuclear weapon that is bought, stolen, or otherwise obtained from a nuclear state, or a weapon fabricated by a terrorist group from illegally obtained fissile nuclear weapons material and produces a nuclear explosion.
INL	Idaho National Laboratory
INS	Incident of national significance
IRB	Institutional Review Board
JFO	Joint field office—The operations of the various federal entities participating in a response at the local level should be collocated in a Joint Field Office whenever possible, to improve the efficiency and effectiveness of federal incident management activities.
JFO-UCG	Unified Coordination Group JFO structure is organized, staffed, and managed in a manner consistent with NIMS principles and is led by the Unified Coordination Group. Personnel from federal and state departments and agencies, other jurisdictional entities, and private sector businesses and NGOs may be requested to staff various levels of the JFO, depending on the requirements of the incident.
JIC	Joint information center—A focal point for the coordination and provision of information to the public and media concerning the federal response to the emergency.

JOC	Joint operations center—The focal point for management and coordination of local, state, and federal investigative/law enforcement activities.
keV	Kiloelectron volts
KI	Potassium iodide
km	Kilometer
LANL	Los Alamos National Laboratory
LBNL	Lawrence Berkely National Laboratory
LFA	Lead Federal Agency
LLNL	Lawrence Livermore National Laboratory
LLW	Low-level waste
LNT	Or LNT model—Linear No-Threshold dose response for which any dose greater than zero has a positive probability of producing an effect (e.g., mutation or cancer). The probability is calculated either from the slope of a linear (L) model or from the limiting slope, as the dose approaches zero, of a linear-quadratic (LQ) model.
LSC	Liquid scintillation counter
m	Meter
mCi	Millicurie
MCL	Maximum contaminant level
MCLG	Maximum contaminant level goal
MERRT	Medical Emergency Radiological Response Team—Provides direct patient treatment; assists and trains local health-care providers in managing, handling, and treating radiation-exposed and contaminated casualties; assesses the impact on human health; and provides consultation and technical advice to local, state, and federal authorities.
MeV	Mega-electron volts or 1E6 eV
mR	Milliroentgen (unit of exposure to x- or gamma-radiation)
mRad	Millirad
MRE	Meals ready to eat
mrem	Millirem (a unit of radiation dose)
N	Number of atoms or depending on context number of neutrons
NaI	Sodium iodide
NaI(Tl)	Sodium iodide thallium activated
NARAC	National Atmospheric Release Advisory Capability
NARM	Nuclear Accelerator-Produced Radioactive Materials
NASA	National Aeronautics and Space Administration
NCC	National Coordinating Center for Telecommunications

nCi	Nanocurie—1nCi = 37 dps or 37 Bq
NCP	National Oil and Hazardous Substances Pollution Contingency Plan (40 CFR part 300)—The Plan provides the organizational structure and procedures for preparing for and responding to discharges of oil and releases of hazardous substances, pollutants, and contaminants.
NCRP	National Council on Radiation Protection and Measurements
NCS	National Communications System
NDA	National Defense Area
NID	Negligible incremental dose
NIEHS	National Institute for Environmental Health Sciences
NIMS	National Incident Management System—The Homeland Security Act of 2002 and HPSD–5 directed the DHS to develop NIMS. The purpose of the NIMS is to provide a consistent, nationwide approach for federal, state, and local governments to work effectively and efficiently together to prepare for, respond to, and recover from domestic incidents.
NIR	Negligible incremental risk
NIRT	Nuclear Incident Response Team—Created by the Homeland Security Act of 2002, the NIRT consists of radiological emergency response assets of the DOE and the EPA. When called on by the Secretary for Homeland Security for actual or threatened radiological incidents, these assets come under the "authority, direction, and control" of the Secretary.
NMDP	National Marrow Donor Program
NNSA/HQ	National Nuclear Security Administration Headquarters
NNSA/NSO	National Nuclear Security Administration Nevada Site Office
NOAA	National Oceanic and Atmospheric Administration
NOC	National Operations Center
NORM	Naturally occurring radioactive materials
NPP	Nuclear power plant
NRC	U.S. Nuclear Regulatory Commission
NRDC	Natural Resources Defense Council
NRF	National Response Framework—The successor to the National Response Plan. The Framework presents the doctrine, principles, and architecture by which our nation prepares for and responds to all hazard disasters across all levels of government and all sectors of communities.
NSA	National Security Area

NTS	Nevada Test Site
ORAU	Oak Ridge Associated Universities
ORISE	Oak Ridge Institute for Science
ORNL	Oak Ridge National Laboratory
ORP	Office of Radiation Protection
OSC	On-Scene Coordinator
OSHA	Occupational Safety and Health Administration, U.S. Department of Labor
PAD	Protective action decision
PAG	Protective action guide—The projected dose to a reference individual, from an accidental or deliberate release of radioactive material at which a specific protective action to reduce or avoid that dose is recommended.
PAO	Public Affairs Officer
PAR	Protective Action Recommendation
PB	Prussian blue
PFO	Principal Federal Official—The PFO will act as the Secretary of Homeland Security's local representative, and he/she will oversee and coordinate federal activities for the incident.
PIO	Public Information Officer—The PIO acts as the communications coordinator or spokesperson within the Incident Command System.
PNNL	Pacific Northwest National Laboratory
PPE	Personal protective equipment
psi	Pounds per square inch
PWR	Pressurized water reactor
R	Roentgen—Measure of exposure in air.
R/N	Radiological or nuclear incident
Rad	Radiation absorbed dose. One rad is equal to an absorbed dose of 100 erg/g or 0.01 J/kg. 1 rad = 0.01 gray (Gy).
RAM	Radioactive materials
RAP	Radiological Assistance Program—A DOE emergency response asset that can rapidly deploy at the request of state or local governments for technical assistance in radiological incidents. RAP teams are a deployable asset of the NIRT.
RCO	Regional Coordinating Office
RDD	Radiological Dispersal Device—Any device that causes the purposeful dissemination of radioactive material, across an area with the intent to cause harm, without a nuclear detonation occurring.

REAC/TS	Radiation Emergency Assistance Center/Training Site—A DOE asset located in Oak Ridge, TN, with technical expertise in medical and health assessment concerning internal and external exposure to radioactive materials. REAC/TS is a deployable asset of the NIRT.
RECP	Regional Emergency Communications Planner
RED	Radiological Exposure Device
Rem	Roentgen Equivalent Man; the conventional unit of radiation dose equivalent. 1 rem = 0.01 sievert (Sv).
REMM	Radiation Event Medical Management—A Web-based algorithm providing just-in-time information for medical responders. It is also useful for education and training. Developed by the Office of Assistant Secretary for Preparedness and Response and the National Library of Medicine. Available at http://www.remm.nlm.gov.
RERT	Radiological Emergency Response Team—An EPA team trained to do environmental sampling and analysis of radionuclides. RERT provides assistance during responses and takes over operation of the FRMAC from the DOE at a point in time after the emergency phase. RERT is a deployable asset of the NIRT.
RHP	Radiation Health Physicist
RME	Reasonable maximum exposure
RMEI	Reasonably maximally exposed individual
RSL	Remote Sensing Laboratory
SCO	State Coordinating Officer
SEO	Senior Energy Official
SFO	Senior FEMA Official
SHARC	Sandia Hazard Assessment Response Capability
SI	International System of Units
SiLi	Lithium drifted silicon—a type of X-ray spectrometer
SNF	Spent Nuclear Fuel
SNL	Sandia National Laboratories
Sr	Strontium
SRNL	Savannah River National Laboratory
SSA	Senior Scientific Advisor
Sv	Sievert; the SI unit of radiation dose equivalent. 1 Sv = 100 rem.
TEDE	Total effective dose equivalent—The sum of the effective dose equivalent from external radiation exposure and the committed effective dose equivalent from internal exposure.

TENORM	Technologically Enhanced Naturally Occurring Radioactive Materials
TLD	Thermoluminescent Dosimeter
USDA U.S.	Department of Agriculture
USDOE-RL	Department of Energy—Richland Operations Office (Hanford)
USDOT	United States Department of Transportation
VA	U.S Department of Veterans Administration
WHO	World Health Organization
WIPP	Waste Isolation Pilot Plant
Z	The number of protons in the nucleus
μCi	Microcuries—1 μCi = 3.7E4 dps or Bq
μCi/m^2	Microcuries per square meter
μR/hr	Microroentgen per hour

APPENDIX C

RADIOLOGICAL TERMS

Source: Dictionary of Radiological Terms; U.S. Dept. of Health & Human Services

A

Absorbed dose: the amount of energy deposited by ionizing radiation in a unit mass of tissue. It is expressed in units of joule per kilogram (J/kg) and called "Gray" (Gy).

Actinides: elements in the periodic table with atomic numbers from 90 to 103 (thorium to lawrencium). Actinides with atomic numbers higher than 92 do not occur naturally but are produced artificially by bombarding other elements with particles. These elements are referred to as *Transuranics* or *TRUs*. Included in this set of elements are neptunium (element 93), plutonium (element 94), americium (element 95), curium (element 96), berkelium (element 97), and californium (element 98).

Activity (radioactivity): the rate of decay of radioactive material expressed as the number of nuclei decaying per second measured in units called becquerels or curies.

Acute exposure: an exposure to radiation that occurred in a matter of minutes rather than over a longer time period. See also **chronic exposure**, **exposure**, and **fractionated exposure**.

Radiation Safety: Protection and Management for Homeland Security and Emergency Response. By L. A. Burchfield
Copyright © 2009 John Wiley & Sons, Inc.

Acute Radiation Syndrome (ARS): ARS is also known as radiation sickness. A person exposed to radiation will develop ARS only if the radiation dose was high, penetrating (e.g., X-rays or gamma rays), encompassed most or all of the body, and was received in a short period of time. Clinical severity of the four subsyndromes of ARS (hematopoietic, cutaneous, gastrointestinal, and neurovascular) will vary with dose and host factors (e.g., young or old age, immunosuppression, and medical comorbidity—especially extensive trauma and burns).

Air burst: a nuclear weapon explosion that is high enough in the air to keep the fireball from touching the ground. Because the fireball does not reach the ground and does not pick up any surface material, the radioactivity in the fallout from an air burst is relatively insignificant compared with a surface burst.

Air kerma: the initial kinetic energy of the primary ionizing particles (photoelectrons, Compton electrons, positron/negatron pairs from photon radiation, and scattered nuclei from fast neutrons) produced by the interaction of the incident uncharged radiation in a small volume of air, when it is irradiated by an X-ray beam. Unit of measure is Gray. See also **kerma**.

ALARA: acronym for "as low as reasonably achievable" means making every reasonable effort to maintain exposures to ionizing radiation as far below the dose limits as practical. This principle is key in radiation protection and safety.

Alpha particles: the nucleus of a helium atom, made up of two neutrons and two protons with a charge of $+2$. Certain radioactive nuclei emit alpha particles. Alpha particles generally carry more energy than gamma rays or beta particles, and they deposit that energy quickly while passing through tissue. Alpha particles can be stopped by a thin layer of light material, such as a sheet of paper, and cannot penetrate the outer, dead layer of skin. Therefore, they do not damage living tissue when outside the body. When alpha-emitting isotopes are inhaled or swallowed, however, they are especially damaging because they transfer relatively large amounts of ionizing energy to living cells. See also **beta particles**, **gamma rays**, **neutron**, and **X-ray**.

Americium (Am): a silvery metal; it is a man-made element whose isotopes Am-231 through Am-249 are all radioactive. Am-241 is formed spontaneously by the beta decay of plutonium-241. Trace quantities of Am-241 are widely used in smoke detectors and as neutron sources in neutron moisture gauges.

Atom: the smallest unit of an element that retain all chemical properties of an element.

Atomic mass: (sometimes referred to as atomic weight) the mass of one mole (6.0221415E23 atoms) of a specific element, expressed in atomic mass units or grams per mole. For example, the atomic number of helium-4 is 2, the atomic mass is 4, and the atomic mass is 4.00026 g/mole.

Atomic mass number: the sum of protons and neutrons in the nucleus of an atom.

Atomic mass unit (amu): 1 amu is equal to one twelfth of the mass of a carbon-12 isotope.

Atomic number: the total number of protons in the nucleus of an atom. The atomic number is used to determine an elements position within the periodic table.

B

Background radiation: a composite of all forms of ionizing radiation from natural sources. Terrestrial and cosmic radiation make up most naturally occurring background radiation.

Becquerel (Bq): A decay rate of one disintegration per second. There are 3.7E10 Bq in one Curie (Ci).

Beta burns: Beta-emitting isotopes that have immediate contact with the skin can cause the skin to shed its outer layers. If exposure to high levels of beta-emitting isotopes persists longer than 1 hour, open sores can occur which in turn provides a pathway for radioactive isotopes to enter the body.

Beta particles: electrons ejected from the nucleus of a radioactive isotope. Although they can be stopped by a thin sheet of aluminum, beta particles can penetrate the dead skin layer, which potentially cause burns. They can pose a serious direct or external radiation threat and can be lethal depending on the amount received. They also pose a serious internal radiation threat if beta-emitting isotopes are ingested or inhaled. See also **alpha particles**, **gamma rays**, **neutron**, and **X-ray**.

Bioassay: a measurement of radioactive materials present inside a person's body via analysis of the person's blood, urine, feces, or sweat.

Biological dosimetry (Biodosimetry): the laboratory or clinical methods used to measure or estimate the dose of ionizing radiation energy absorbed by an individual. Biodosimetry tools measure the dose to internal organs and tissues from external exposure and internal contamination.

Biological Effects of Ionizing Radiation (BEIR) Reports: reports of the National Research Council's committee on the Biological Effects of Ionizing Radiation.

Biological half-life: the time required for one half of the amount of a radio-nuclide to be expelled from the body by natural metabolic processes, not counting radioactive decay, once it has been taken in through inhalation, ingestion, or absorption. See also **radioactive half-life** and **effective half-life**.

Burn: the partial or complete destruction of skin caused by some form of energy, usually thermal energy.

C

Carcinogen: a cancer-causing substance.

Cesium-137 (Cs-137): has a half-life of 30.17 years and decays by beta and gamma radiation. Cs-137 is a fission product. It is often used in medical devices and gauges. Small quantities of Cs-137 can be found in the environment from nuclear weapons tests that occurred in the 1950s and 1960s and from nuclear reactor accidents, such as the Chernobyl accident in 1986, which distributed Cs-137 to many countries in Europe.

Chain reaction: a process that initiates its own repetition. In a fission chain reaction, a fissile nucleus absorbs a neutron and fissions (splits) spontaneously, which releases two or three more neutrons. These, in turn, can be absorbed by other fissile nuclei, which release still more neutrons. A fission chain reaction is self-sustaining when the number of neutrons released in a given time equals or exceeds the number of neutrons lost by absorption in nonfissile material or by escape from the system.

Chronic exposure: exposure to a substance over a long period of time, which possibly results in adverse health effects. See also **acute exposure** and **fractionated exposure**.

Cobalt (Co): a gray, hard, magnetic, and somewhat malleable metal. Cobalt is relatively rare and generally obtained as a byproduct of the production of other metals, such as copper. Its most common radioisotope, cobalt-60 (Co-60), is used in radiography and medical applications. Co-60 emits beta particles and gamma rays during radioactive decay.

Collective dose: the estimated dose for an area or region multiplied by the estimated population in that area or region.

Combined injury: physical, thermal, and/or chemical trauma combined with radiation exposure at a dose sufficient to diminish the likelihood of overall survival or functional recovery.

Committed dose: a dose that accounts for continuing exposures expected to be received over a long period of time (such as 30, 50, or 70 years) from radioactive materials that were deposited inside the body.

Conference of Radiation Control Program Directors (CRCPD): an organization whose members represent state radiation protection programs.

Contamination (radioactive): the deposition of unwanted radioactive material
on the surfaces of structures, areas, objects, or people where it may be external
or internal. See also decontamination and incorporation. Contamination
means that radioactive materials in the form of gases, liquids, or solids are
released into the environment and contaminate people externally, internally,
or both. An external surface of the body, such as the skin, can become
contaminated, and if radioactive materials get inside the body through the
lungs, gut, or wounds, the contaminant can become deposited internally.

Controlled area: an area where entry, activities, and exit are controlled to help
ensure radiation protection and prevent the spread of contamination.

Cosmic radiation: radiation produced in outer space when heavy particles
(nuclei of all known natural elements) bombard the earth. See also **background radiation** and **terrestrial radiation**.

Criticality: a fission process where the neutron production rate equals the
neutron loss rate to absorption or leakage. A nuclear reactor is said to be
"critical" when it is operating.

Critical mass: the minimum amount of fissile material that can achieve a
self-sustaining nuclear chain reaction.

Cumulative dose: the total dose that results from repeated or continuous
exposures of the same portion of the body, or of the whole body, to ionizing
radiation.

Curie (Ci): the curie was defined originally as the observed decay rate of 1 g
of radium. Today, one curie of radioactive material produces exactly 37 billion disintegrations in 1 second.

Cutaneous Radiation Syndrome (CRS): the complex syndrome that results
from radiation exposure of more than 200 rads to the skin. The immediate
effects can be reddening and swelling of the exposed area (like a severe
burn), blisters, ulcers on the skin, hair loss, and severe pain. Very large
doses can result in permanent hair loss, scarring, altered skin color, deterio-
ration of the affected body part, and death of the affected tissue (requiring
surgery).

D

Decay chain or decay series: There are only three naturally occurring decay
series: thorium, uranium, and actinium. The beginning isotope for the thorium series (4N + 0 series) is Th-232, which decays through 10 daughter isotopes that decay to Pb-208. The beginning isotope for the uranium series

(4N + 2 series) is U-238, which in turn decays through 13 daughter isotopes (excluding minor daughters) and that decays to Pb-206. The beginning isotope for the actinium series (4N + 3) is U-235, which decays through 10 daughter isotopes (excluding minor daughters) and decays to Pb-207.

Decay products or daughter products: the isotopes formed during radioactive decay. Also known as "decay chain products" or "progeny." A decay product may be either radioactive or stable.

Decay, radioactive: disintegration of an unstable nucleus by the release of radiation in the form of electromagnetic or particles directly from the nucleus.

Decay rate constant: the fraction of nuclear decays occurring in a unit of time. The decay rate constant is inversely proportional to the radioactive half-life.

Decontamination (radioactive): the reduction or removal of radioactive contamination from a structure, object, or person.

Decorporation: removal of radioactive isotopes from the body using specific drugs called "decorporation agents."

Depleted uranium: uranium that contains less than 0.7% uranium-235, the amount found in natural uranium. See also **enriched uranium**.

Deposition density: the activity of a radionuclide deposited per unit area of ground. Generally reported as becquerels per square meter or curies per square meter.

Detector: A device that is sensitive to radiation and can produce a response signal suitable for measurement or analysis. A radiation detection instrument.

Deterministic effect: an effect that can be related directly to the radiation dose received. The severity increases as the dose increases. A deterministic effect typically has a threshold below which the effect will not occur. See also **stochastic effect** and **nonstochastic effect**.

Deuterium: a nonradioactive isotope of the hydrogen atom that contains a neutron in its nucleus in addition to the one proton normally observed in hydrogen. A deuterium atom is twice as heavy as normal hydrogen. See also **tritium**.

Dirty bomb: a device designed to spread radioactive material by conventional explosives when the bomb explodes. A dirty bomb kills or injures people through the initial blast of the conventional explosive and spreads radioactive contamination over possibly a large area—hence, the term "dirty." Such bombs could be miniature devices or large truck bombs. A dirty bomb is much simpler to make than a true nuclear weapon. See also radiological dispersal device. It should also be pointed out that this term has evolved over time. In the 1960s, a dirty bomb was meant to be a nuclear weapon that was built with cobalt. Such a device would "activate" the stable cobalt into radioactive cobalt which in turn would cause much more damage from the highly radioactive Co-60.

Dose (radiation): radiation absorbed by a person's body. Several different terms describe radiation dose. See **rem**, **rad**, **sievert**, and **gray**.

Dose coefficient: the factor used to convert radionuclide intake to dose. Usually expressed as dose per unit intake (e.g., sieverts per becquerel).

Dose equivalent: a quantity used in radiation protection to place all radiation on a common scale for calculating tissue damage. Dose equivalent is the absorbed dose in grays multiplied by a quality factor. The quality factor accounts for differences in radiation effects caused by different types of ionizing radiation. Some radiation, including alpha particles, causes a greater amount of damage per unit of absorbed dose than other radiation. The sievert (Sv) is the unit used to measure dose equivalent.

Dose rate: the radiation dose delivered per unit of time.

Dose reconstruction: a scientific study that estimates doses to people from releases of radioactivity or other pollutants. The dose is reconstructed by determining the amount of material released, the way people came in contact with it, and the amount they absorbed.

Dosimeter: a small portable instrument [such as a film badge, thermoluminescent dosimeter (TLD), or pocket dosimeter] for measuring and recording the total accumulated dose of ionizing radiation a person receives.

Dosimetry: assessment (by measurement or calculation) of radiation dose.

E

Effective dose: a quantity useful for comparing the overall health affects of irradiation of the whole body. It takes into account the absorbed doses received by various organs and tissues and weighs them according to present knowledge of the sensitivity of each organ to radiation. It also accounts for the type of radiation and the potential for each type to inflict biologic damage. The effective dose is used, for example, to compare the overall health detriments of different radionuclides in a given mix. The unit of effective dose is the sievert (Sv); $1 \, Sv = 1 \, J/kg$.

Effective half-life: the time required for the amount of a radionuclide deposited in a living organism to be diminished by 50% as a result of the combined action of radioactive decay and biological elimination. See also **biological half-life**, **decay constant**, and **radioactive half-life**.

Electromagnetic radiation: Generally, the public refers to light as "visible light." Physicists, however, refer to the light as the entire electromagnetic spectrum. Types of electromagnetic radiation range from those of short wavelength, like X-rays and gamma rays, through the ultraviolet, visible, and infrared regions, to radar and radio waves of relatively long wavelengths. All forms of the electromagnetic spectrum travel at the same speed (the speed of light—299792458 m/s) in a vacuum. Individual packets of light are referred to as photons. Photons that originate from the nucleus are referred to as gamma radiation, regardless of its energy. Likewise, photons that originate from inner shell electrons of the atom are referred to as X-rays. Generally, X-rays possess energies from about 0.5 keV to approximately 110 keV. Gamma rays possess energies from approximately 20 KeV to 30 MeV.

Electron: an elementary particle with a negative electrical charge and a mass 1/1836 that of the proton. Electrons surround the nucleus of an atom because of the attraction between their negative charge and the positive charge of the nucleus. A stable atom will have as many electrons as it has protons. See also **neutron**.

Electron volt (eV): a unit of energy equivalent to the amount of energy gained by an electron when it passes from a point of low potential to a point one volt higher in potential.

Element: (1) all isotopes of an atom that contain the same number of protons. For example, the element uranium has 92 protons, and the different isotopes of this element may contain 126 to 150 neutrons. (2) In a reactor, a fuel element is a metal rod that contains the fissile material.

Enriched uranium: uranium in which the proportion of the isotope uranium-235 has been increased by physically removing uranium-238. See also **depleted uranium**.

Epidemiology: the study of the distribution and determinants of health-related states or events in specified populations, and the application of this study to the control of health problems.

Exposure pathway: a route by which a radionuclide or other toxic material can enter the body. The main exposure routes are inhalation, ingestion, absorption through the skin, and entry through a cut or wound in the skin.

Exposure (radiation): a general term used loosely to express what a person receives as a result of being exposed to ionizing radiation.

Exposure rate: the amount of ionization produced per unit time in air by X-rays or gamma rays. The unit of exposure rate is Roentgens/hour (R/hr); for decommissioning activities the typical units are microRoentgens per hour (μR/hr), i.e., 10^{-6} R/hr.

External irradiation (or external exposure): external irradiation occurs when all or part of the body is exposed to penetrating radiation from an external source. During exposure, this radiation can be absorbed by the body or it can pass completely through. An example would be an ordinary chest

X-ray. Following external exposure, an individual is not radioactive and can be treated like any other patient. Gamma or photon radiation exposure from a terrorist nuclear event or radiation dispersal device would make the victim at risk for acute radiation syndrome, depending on the dose received.

F

Fallout, nuclear: fission products (from a nuclear bomb) that have condensed onto minute particles that descend slowly from the atmosphere after a nuclear explosion. Generally, nuclear fallout is associated with an above-ground nuclear detonation releasing debris into the open atmosphere.

Fissile material: any material in which neutrons can cause a fission reaction. The three primary fissile materials are uranium-233, uranium-235, and plutonium-239.

Fission (fissioning): the splitting of a nucleus into at least two other nuclei that releases a large amount of energy. Two or three neutrons are usually released during this transformation. See also **fusion**.

Fractionated exposure: exposure to radiation that occurs in several small acute exposures, rather than continuously as in a chronic exposure.

Fusion: a reaction in which at least one heavier, more stable nucleus is produced from two lighter, less-stable nuclei. Reactions of this type are responsible for the release of energy in stars or in thermonuclear devices.

G

Gamma rays: high-energy electromagnetic radiation emitted by certain radionuclides when their nuclei transition from a higher to a lower energy state. These rays have high energy and a short wavelength. All gamma rays emitted from a given isotope have the same energy; this characteristic enables scientists to identify specific isotopes. Gamma rays penetrate tissue farther than do beta or alpha particles but leave a lower concentration of ions in their path potentially to cause cell damage. All gamma rays are emitted from the nucleus. X-rays, however, are emitted when an inner shell electron is ejected from an atom.

Geiger counter: a radiation detection and measuring instrument that consists of a gas-filled tube containing electrodes, between which an electrical voltage but no current flows. When ionizing radiation passes through the tube, a short, intense pulse of current passes from the negative electrode to the positive electrode and is measured or counted. The number of pulses per second measures the intensity of the radiation field. Geiger counters are the most commonly used portable radiation detection instruments.

Generator: a long-term power source for remote equipment, such as light-houses on Russia's Arctic coast or U.S. unmanned space probes. Typical isotopes used include strontium-90, cesium-137, and plutonium-238.

Genetic effects: hereditary effects (mutations) that can be passed on through reproduction because of mutations in the DNA or RNA. See also **teratogenic effects** and **somatic effects**.

Gray (Gy): the new International System (SI) unit of radiation dose, which is expressed as absorbed energy per unit mass of tissue. The SI unit "Gray" has replaced the older "rad" designation. (1 Gy = 1 joule/kilogram = 100 rad). Gray can be used for any type of radiation (e.g., alpha, beta, neutron, or gamma), but it does not describe the biological effects of different radiations. Biological effects of radiation are measured in units of "Sievert" (or the older designation "rem"). Sievert is calculated as follows: Gray multiplied by the "radiation weighting factor" (also known as the "quality factor") associated with a specific type of radiation.

H

Half-life: the time any substance takes to decay by half of its original amount. See also **biological half-life**, **decay constant**, **effective half-life**, and **radioactive half-life**.

Health physics: a scientific field that focuses on protection of humans and the environment from radiation. Health physics uses physics, biology, chemistry, statistics, and electronic instrumentation to help protect individuals from any damaging effects of radiation. For more information, see the Health Physics Society website at http://www.hps.org/.

High-level radioactive waste: the radioactive material that results from spent nuclear fuel reprocessing. This material can include liquid waste directly produced in reprocessing or any solid material derived from the liquid waste having a sufficient concentration of fission. Other radioactive materials can be designated as high-level waste if they require permanent isolation. This determination is made by the U.S. Nuclear Regulatory Commission on the basis of criteria established in U.S. law. See also **low-level waste** and **transuranic waste**.

Highly enriched uranium (HEU): uranium that is enriched to above 20% uranium-235 (U-235). Weapons-grade HEU is enriched to above 90% in U-235.

Hot spot: any place where the level of radioactive contamination is considerably greater than the area around it.

I

Incorporation: refers to the uptake of radioactive materials by body cells, tissues, and target organs, such as bone, liver, thyroid, or kidney. In general, radioactive materials are distributed throughout the body based on their chemical properties. Incorporation cannot occur unless contamination has occurred. Incorporation is also called internal contamination, (REAC/TS).

Ingestion: (1) the act of swallowing. (2) In the case of radionuclides or chemicals, swallowing radionuclides or chemicals by eating or drinking.

Inhalation: (1) the act of breathing in. (2) In the case of radionuclides or chemicals, breathing in radionuclides or chemicals.

Internal exposure: exposure to radioactive material taken into the body.

Inverse square law: the relationship that states that radiation intensity is inversely proportional to the square of the distance from a point source.

Iodine: a nonmetallic solid element. Both radioactive and stable isotopes of iodine exist. Radioactive isotopes of iodine are widely used in medical applications. Radioiodine is a biological "getter" because stable iodine is an essential element to life. Radioactive iodine is a volatile fission product and is generally considered to be the largest contributor to people's radiation dose after an accident at a nuclear reactor. Exposure to radioiodine can be reduced by taking so-called "radiation pills." These pills contain nothing more than stable sodium or potassium iodide. By "flooding" the body with stable iodine, the body is less likely to have an uptake of radioiodine.

Ion: an atom that has fewer or more electrons than it has protons, which causes it to have an electrical charge and, therefore, form either a cation (positive ion) or an anion (negative ion).

Ionization: the process of adding one or more electrons to, or removing one or more electrons from, atoms or molecules, which thereby creates ions. High temperatures, electrical discharges, or nuclear radiation can cause ionization.

Ionizing radiation: any radiation that can displace electrons from atoms, which thereby produces ions. High doses of ionizing radiation may produce severe skin or tissue damage. See also **alpha particles**, **beta particles**, **gamma rays**, **neutron**, and **X-ray**.

Iridium-192: a gamma-ray-emitting radioisotope used for gamma radiography. The half-life is 73.827 days.

Irradiation: exposure to radiation.

Irradiator: large device that sterilizes food, medical equipment, or blood for transfusion. Irradiators are even used to enhance color in gemstones; examples include cobalt-60 or cesium-137.

Isotope: a nuclide of an element that has the same number of protons but a different number of neutrons.

K

Kerma: the initial kinetic energy of the primary ionizing particles (photoelectrons, Compton electrons, positron/negatron pairs from photon radiation, and scattered nuclei from fast neutrons) produced by the interaction of the incident uncharged radiation, per unit mass of interacting medium. The unit of measure is gray. See also **air kerma**.

Kiloton (Kt): the energy of an explosion that is equivalent to an explosion of 1000 tons of TNT. One kiloton equals 1 trillion (1E12) calories. See also **megaton**.

L

Latent period: the time between exposure to a toxic material and the appearance of a resultant health effect.

Lead (Pb): a heavy metal. Lead has the highest atomic number of any element containing stable isotopes. Lead has four stable isotopes (204, 206, 207, and 208) and 33 radioactive isotopes. Many of the radioactive isotopes of lead, such as Pb-210 are beta emitters and are naturally present in the thorium, uranium, and actinium decay chains.

Lead federal agency (LFA): the federal agency that leads and coordinates the emergency response activities of other federal agencies during a nuclear emergency. After a nuclear emergency, the Federal Radiological Emergency Response Plan (FRERP, available at http://www.fas.org/nuke/guide/usa/doctrine/national/frerp.htm) will determine which federal agency will be the LFA.

Lethal dose (50/30): the dose of radiation expected to cause death within 30 days to 50% of those exposed without medical treatment. The generally accepted dose is about 400 rem received over a short period of time.

Local radiation injury (LRI): acute radiation exposure (more than 1000 rads) to a small, localized part of the body. Most local radiation injuries do not cause death. However, if the exposure is from penetrating radiation (neutrons, X-rays, or gamma rays), internal organs may be damaged, and some symptoms of ARS, which includes death, may occur. Local radiation injury invariably involves skin damage, and a skin graft or other surgery may be required.

Low-level waste (LLW): radioactively contaminated industrial or research waste, such as paper, rags, plastic bags, medical waste, and water-treatment residues. It is waste that does not meet the criteria for any of three other categories of radioactive waste, which includes spent nuclear fuel and high-level radioactive waste, transuranic waste, or uranium mill tailings. Its categorization does not depend on the level of radioactivity it contains.

M

Megaton (Mt): the energy of an explosion that is equivalent to an explosion of 1 million tons of TNT. One megaton is equal to a quintillion (1E18) calories. See also **kiloton**.

Monitoring: determining the amount of ionizing radiation or radioactive contamination present. Also referred to as surveying.

N

Neoplastic: pertaining to the pathologic process that results in the formation and growth of an abnormal mass of tissue.

Neutron: a small subatomic particle possessing no electrical charge, typically found within an atom's nucleus. Neutrons are, as the name implies, neutral in their charge. A neutron has about the same mass as a proton. See also **alpha particles**, **beta particles**, **gamma rays**, **nucleon**, and **X-ray**.

Nonionizing radiation: radiation that has lower energy levels than ionizing radiation. Nonionizing radiation does not possess enough energy to impact the structure of atoms it contacts, but it does possess enough energy to heat tissue and can cause harmful biological effects. Examples include radio waves, microwaves, visible light, and infrared from a heat lamp.

Nonstochastic effect: an effect that can be related directly to the radiation dose received. The effect is more severe with a higher dose. It typically has a threshold, below which the effect will not occur. It is sometimes called deterministic effect. For example, a skin burn from radiation is a nonstochastic effect that worsens as the radiation dose increases. See also **stochastic effect**.

Nuclear energy: the heat energy produced by the process of nuclear fission within a nuclear reactor or by radioactive decay.

Nuclear fuel cycle: the steps involved in supplying fuel for nuclear power plants. It can include mining, milling, isotopic enrichment, fabrication of fuel elements, use in reactors, chemical reprocessing to recover the fissile material remaining in the spent fuel, reenrichment of the fuel material refabrication into new fuel elements, and waste disposal.

Nuclear reactor: a device in which a controlled, self-sustaining nuclear chain reaction can be maintained with the use of cooling to remove generated heat.

Nuclear (radioactive) tracers: All isotopes of the same element behave chemically the same. This principle implies that if a radioactive isotope (tracer) is substituted for a stable isotope, then the chemical or biological process can be followed by measuring the radioactive decay of the tracer.

Nucleon: currently protons and neutrons can not be distinguished while they remain in the nucleus. As a result, both are not distinguished and each are referred to as nucleons.

Nucleus: the central part of an atom that contains protons and neutrons. The nucleus is 100,000 times smaller than the atom. The atom is 99.999% empty space, and the nucleus makes up 99.99% of an atoms mass.

Nuclide: a general term applicable to all isotopes. Nuclides are identified by the elemental chemical symbol and their atomic mass number. For example—Sr-90 is a radioactive *nuclide* that contains 38 protons (atomic number 38) and 52 neutrons ($90 - 32 = 52$).

P

Pathways: the routes by which people are exposed to radiation or other contaminants. The four basic pathways are inhalation, ingestion, puncture wounds, and direct external exposure. See also **exposure pathway**.

Penetrating radiation: radiation that can penetrate the skin and reach internal organs and internal tissues. Energetic photons (such as gamma rays and X-rays), neutrons, and protons are forms of penetrating radiation. However, alpha particles and all but extremely high-energy beta particles are not considered penetrating radiation.

Photon: a discrete "packet" of pure electromagnetic energy. Photons have no mass and travel at the speed of light. The term "photon" was developed to describe energy when it acts like a particle (causing interactions at the molecular or atomic level) rather than a wave. Gamma rays and X-rays are both types photons.

Pitchblende: a brown to black mineral that has a distinctive luster. It consists mainly of uraninite (UO_2), but it also contains radium (Ra). It is the main source of uranium (U) ore.

Plume: a specific type of environmental contaminant or material that spreads from a particular source and travels through environmental media, such as air or ground water. For example, a plume could describe the dispersal of particles, gases, vapors, and aerosols in the atmosphere, or the movement of contamination through an aquifer (such as through dilution, mixing, or adsorption onto soil).

Plutonium (Pu): a heavy, man-made, radioactive metallic element. The most important isotope is Pu-239, which has a half-life of 24,000 years. Pu-239 can be used in reactor fuel and is a primary fissile material used in nuclear weapons. One kilogram of Pu-239 can release an equivalent of about 22 million kwh of heat energy either from a nuclear weapon or in a nuclear reactor. In the detonation of a nuclear weapon, a kilogram of plutonium will produce an explosion that is equal to approximately 20,000 tons of chemical explosive. All isotopes of plutonium are readily absorbed by the bones, and it has a biological life (once absorbed by bones) of approximately 85 years.

Polonium (Po): a radioactive element that is found as a daughter product in all three naturally occurring decay chains (thorium, uranium, and actinium). Po-210 fell into the public spot light after being used to poison Alexander Litvinenko (a former KGB agent) in November 2006. By mass, polonium-210 is around 250,000 times more toxic than hydrogen cyanide (the actual LD50 for 210Po is about 1 μg for an 80-kg person).

Prenatal radiation exposure: radiation exposure to an embryo or fetus while it is still in its mother's womb. At certain stages of the pregnancy, the fetus is particularly sensitive to radiation and the health consequences could be severe above 5 rads, especially to brain function.

Protective action guide (PAG): a guide that tells state and local authorities at what projected dose they should take action to protect people from exposure to unplanned releases of radioactive material into the environment.

Proton: a small subatomic particle found in the nucleus of all atoms. Protons that possesses a positive electrical charge of $+1$. Even though protons are about 1836 times heavier than electrons, they are approximately 100,000 times smaller than an atom. The number of protons is unique for each chemical element. See also **nucleon**.

Q

Quality factor (Q): the factor by which the absorbed dose (rad or gray) is multiplied to obtain a quantity that expresses, on a common scale for all ionizing radiation, the biological damage (rem) to an exposed person. It is used because some types of radiation, such as alpha particles, are more biologically damaging internally than other types.

Radiation weighting factors from ICRP Publication 60 (ICRP 1991):

Type of Radiation	Quality Factor
Photons, all energies	1
Electrons and muons, all energies	1
Neutrons, energies less than 10 keV	5
10 keV to 100 keV	10
100 keV to 2 MeV	20
2 MeV to 20 MeV	10
Energies greater than 20 MeV	5
Protons, energies greater than 2 MeV	5
Alpha particles, fission fragments, and heavy nuclei	20

R

Rad (radiation absorbed dose): a basic unit of absorbed radiation dose. It is a measure of the amount of energy absorbed by the body. The rad was the original unit of absorbed dose. It has been replaced by the unit gray (Gy), which is equivalent to 100 rad. One rad equals the dose delivered to an object of 100 ergs of energy per gram of material.

Radiation: energy that moves in the form of particles or waves. Familiar radiations are heat, light, radio waves, and microwaves. Ionizing radiation is a very high-energy form of radiation that causes matter to become ionized.

Radiation sickness: See also **acute radiation syndrome (ARS)**.

Radioactive contamination: the deposition of unwanted radioactive material on the surfaces of structures, areas, objects, or people. It can be airborne, external, or internal. See also **contamination** and **decontamination**.

Radioactive decay: the spontaneous disintegration of the nucleus of an atom.

Radioactive half-life: the time required for a quantity of a radioisotope to decay by half. For example, because the half-life of iodine-131 (I-131) is 8 days, a sample of I-131 that has 10 mCi of activity on January 1, will have 5 mCi of activity 8 days later, on January 9. See also **biological half-life**, **decay constant**, and **effective half-life**.

Radioactive material: material that contains unstable (radioactive) nuclei that give off radiation as they decay.

Radioactivity: the process of spontaneous transformation of the nucleus, generally with the emission of alpha or beta particles or gamma rays. This process is referred to as decay or disintegration of an atom.

Radioactive waste: disposable, radioactive materials that result from nuclear operations. Wastes are generally classified into the following categories: high-level, mixed, and low-level waste.

Radioassay: both qualitative and quantitative analysis to determine the amounts of radioactive materials through the detection of ionizing radiation. Radioassays will detect transuranic nuclides, uranium, fission and activation products, naturally occurring radioactive material, and medical isotopes.

Radiogenic: health effects caused by exposure to ionizing radiation.

Radiography: (1) *medical:* the use of radiant energy (such as X-rays and gamma rays) to image body systems. (2) *Industrial:* the use of radioactive sources to photograph internal structures, such as turbine blades in jet engines. A sealed radiation source, usually iridium-192 (Ir-192) or cobalt-60 (Co-60), used to produce beams of gamma rays to interrogate objects or people. For example, gamma rays that pass through flaws in the metal or incomplete welds strike special photographic film (radiographic film) on the opposite side and thus demonstrate flaws.

Radioisotope (radioactive isotope): isotopes of an element that have an unstable nucleus. Radioactive isotopes are commonly used in science, industry, and medicine. A radioactive isotope will eventually decay to a stable isotope through one or more radioactive decays. Approximately 3700 natural and artificial radioisotopes have been identified.

Radiological or radiologic: related to radioactive materials or radiation. The radiological sciences focus on the measurement and effects of radiation.

Radioluminescence: the luminescence produced by particles emitted during radioactive decay.

Radiological dispersal device (RDD): a device that disperses radioactive material by conventional explosive or other mechanical means, such as a spray. See also dirty bomb.

Radiological exposure device (RED): also called a "hidden sealed source." An RED is a terrorist device intended to expose people to significant doses of ionizing radiation without their knowledge. Constructed from partially or fully unshielded radioactive material, an RED could be hidden from sight in a public place (e.g., under a subway seat, in a food court, or in a busy hallway), exposing those who sit or pass close by.

If the seal around the source were broken and the radioactive contents released from the container, the device could become an RDD, which can cause radiological contamination.

Radionuclide: an unstable and therefore radioactive form of a nuclide or isotope.

Radiotherapy: external-beam treatment or internal implanting of radioactive isotopes for medical therapy.

Radium (Ra): a naturally occurring radioactive metal. Radium is a radionuclide formed by the decay of uranium (U) and thorium (Th) in the environment. It occurs at low levels in virtually all rocks, soil, water, plants, and animals. Radon (Rn) is a decay product of radium.

Radon (Rn): a naturally occurring radioactive gas found in soil, rock, and water throughout the United States. Radon may cause lung cancer and is a threat to health because it tends to collect in homes, sometimes to very high concentrations. As a result, radon is the largest source of exposure to people from naturally occurring radiation.

Relative risk: the ratio between the risk for disease in an irradiated population to the risk in an unexposed population. A relative risk of 1:1 indicates a 10% increase in cancer from radiation, compared with the "normal" incidence. See also **risk**.

Relative biologic effectiveness (RBE): The RBE of some test radiation (r) compared with X-rays is defined by the ratio D250/Dr, where D250 and Dr, respectively, are the doses of X-rays and the test radiation required for equal biologic effect. (National Bureau of Standards, 1954)

Rem (roentgen equivalent, man): a unit of equivalent dose. Not all radiation has the same biological effect, even for the same amount of absorbed dose. Rem relates the absorbed dose in human tissue to the effective biological damage of the radiation. It is determined by multiplying the number of rads by the quality factor; a this number reflects the potential damage caused by the particular type of radiation. The rem is the traditional unit of equivalent dose, but it is being replaced by the sievert (Sv), which is equal to 100 rem.

Risk: the probability of injury, disease, or death under specific circumstances and time periods. Risk can be expressed as a value that ranges from 0% (no injury or harm will occur) to 100% (harm or injury will definitely occur). Risk can be influenced by several factors: personal behavior or lifestyle, environmental exposure to other material, or an inborn or inherited characteristic known from scientific evidence to be associated with a health effect. Because many risk factors are not exactly measurable, the risk estimates are uncertain. See also **relative risk**.

Risk assessment: an evaluation of the risk to human health or the environment by hazards. Risk assessments can examine at either existing hazards or potential hazards.

Roentgen (R): a unit of exposure to X-rays or gamma rays. One roentgen is the amount of gamma or X-rays needed to produce ions that carry 1 electrostatic unit of electrical charge in 1 cm^3 of dry air under standard conditions.

S

Sealed source: A radioactive source sealed in an impervious container that has sufficient mechanical strength to prevent contact with and dispersion of the radioactive material under the conditions of use and wear for which it was designed. Generally used for radiography or radiation therapy. May be classified "Special Form" on shipping papers and packages.

Sensitivity (to radioactivity): ability of an analytical method to detect small concentrations of radioactive material.

Shielding: the material between a radiation source and the environment or personnel.

Sievert (Sv): a unit used to derive a quantity called dose equivalent. This relates the absorbed dose in human tissue to the effective biological damage of the radiation. Not all radiation has the same biological effect, even for the same amount of absorbed dose. Dose equivalent is often expressed as millionths of a sievert, or microsieverts (μSv). One sievert is equivalent to 100 rem.

Somatic effects: effects of radiation that are limited to the exposed person, as distinguished from genetic effects, which may also affect subsequent generations. See also **teratogenic effects**.

Stable nucleus: a nucleus that does not undergo nuclear decay. See also **unstable nucleus**.

Special Nuclear Material (SNM): plutonium and uranium enriched in the isotope uranium-233 or uranium-235.

Stochastic effect: an effect that occurs on a random basis independent of the size of the dose. The effect typically has no threshold and is based on probabilities, with the chances of seeing the effect increasing with dose. If it occurs, the severity of a stochastic effect is independent of the dose received. Cancer is a stochastic effect. See also **nonstochastic effect** and **deterministic effect**.

Strontium (Sr): a silvery, soft metal that rapidly turns yellow in air. Sr-90 is a fission product. Approximately 6% of all fission events yield Sr-90. Sr-90 emits beta particles during radioactive decay (with no gammas), and it is one of the few fission products that does not emit both beta and gammas.

Surface burst: a nuclear weapon explosion that is close enough to the ground for the radius of the fireball to vaporize surface material. Fallout from a surface burst contains very high levels of radioactivity. See also **air burst**.

T

Tailings: waste rock from mining operations that contains concentrations of mineral ore that are too low to make typical extraction methods economical.

Teratogenic effects: birth defects that are not passed on to future generations, which are caused by exposure to a toxin as a fetus. See also **genetic effects** and **somatic effects**.

Terrestrial radiation: radiation emitted by naturally occurring radioactive materials, such as uranium (U), thorium (Th), and radon (Rn) in the earth.

Thermonuclear device: a "hydrogen bomb." A device with explosive energy that comes from fusion of small nuclei, as well as from fission.

Thorium (Th): a naturally occurring radioactive metal found in small amounts in soil, rock, water, plants, and animals. The most common isotopes of thorium are thorium-232 (Th-232), thorium-230 (Th-230), and thorium-238 (Th-238).

Total Effective Dose Equivalent (TEDE): The sum of an effective dose equivalent from external radiation and the committed effective dose equivalent from inhaled and ingested radioactive material. Quoted in units of rem.

Transuranic (TRUs): pertaining to elements with atomic numbers higher than uranium (92). For example, plutonium (Pu) and americium (Am) are transuranics.

Tritium: (symbol H-3) a radioactive isotope of the element hydrogen (chemical symbol H). See also deuterium. Tritium, deuterium, and hydrogen are the only isotopes with formal names.

U

UNSCEAR: United Nations Scientific Committee on the Effects of Atomic Radiation. See also http://www.unscear.org/.

Unstable nucleus: a nucleus that disintegrates through radioactive decay (i.e., the nucleus of a radioactive isotope). See also **stable nucleus**.

Uranium (U): a naturally occurring radioactive element whose principal isotopes are uranium-238 (U-238), uranium-235 (U-235), and uranium-234 (U-234). Natural uranium is a hard, silvery-white, shiny metallic ore that contains all three of the above-listed isotopes.

Uranium mill tailings: naturally radioactive residue from the processing of uranium ore. Although the milling process recovers about 95% of the uranium, the residues, or tailings, contain several isotopes of naturally occurring radioactive material, which includes uranium (U), thorium (Th), radium (Ra), polonium (Po), and radon (Rn).

W

Whole-body count: the measure and analysis of the radiation being emitted from a person's entire body, which is detected by a counter external to the body.

Whole-body exposure: an exposure of the body to radiation, in which the entire body, rather than an isolated part, is irradiated by an external source.

X

X-ray: electromagnetic radiation caused by removal of electrons from inner orbitals of an atom. X-rays, like gamma rays, can travel long distances through air and most other materials. Like gamma rays, X-rays require more shielding to reduce their intensity than do beta or alpha particles. X-rays and gamma rays differ primarily in their origin: X-rays originate in the inner shell electrons; gamma rays originate in the nucleus. See also **neutron**. X-rays possess energies between 0.5 keV and approximately 110 keV.

APPENDIX D

RADIOLOGICAL ATTACK— RADIOLOGICAL DISPERSAL DEVICES— INCIDENT PLANNING GUIDE

State of California Hospital Incident Command System—External Scenarios

The Universal Adversary terrorist group detonates a radiological dispersal device (RDD), or "dirty bomb," containing cesium chloride in your city. Approximately a 36-block area is severely damaged and is contaminated with low levels of radiation. The bomb blast injures a large number of people, some with fragment wounds with radiological material imbedded. There are multiple fatalities. The first emergency medical service (EMS) and fire responders into the scene are contaminated with low levels of radiation, but quickly a secure perimeter and triage/decontamination areas are established in the primary impact area.

Your hospital is located 5 miles from the blast zone, and the explosion did not disrupt utilities (power, water, and communications) to your facility. The local emergency operations center (EOC), however, was impacted by the blast as it was located within the 36-block area.

Your hospital is notified of the bomb blast and the possible radiological contamination, and you immediately prepare for contaminated victims that will self-present at the facility without field decontamination.

Radiation Safety: Protection and Management for Homeland Security and Emergency Response. By L. A. Burchfield
Copyright © 2009 John Wiley & Sons, Inc.

Does your Emergency Management Plan Address the following issues?

Mitigation and Preparedness

1. Does your hospital have a procedure securing the facility and controlling access and egress?

2. Does your security department receive regular training on managing facility security and personal protection during a radioactive event?

3. Does your hospital have a plan for decontamination of radiologically contaminated victims, including monitoring of staff and decontamination of the facility?

4. Does your hospital train staff on radiological emergencies, including the appropriate level and type of personal protective equipment required?

5. Does your hospital have a process to determine the safety threat to your facility from the radiological dispersal device blast and whether you need to shelter-in-place?

6. Does your hospital have a procedure to obtain incident specific details from the emergency management agency and/or local emergency operations center (EOC)?

7. Does your hospital have a procedure for detecting for and monitoring radiation levels in the facility and in people? If not, who would you contact to provide this service if needed?

Response and Recovery

1. Does your hospital have radiological response and victim decontamination plan?

2. Does your hospital have a plan to implement radiological monitoring and detection for staff, patients, and visitors?

3. Does your hospital have a protocol and criteria for determining shelter-in-place and/or evacuation of the facility is needed?

4. Does your hospital have a procedure to provide appropriate personal protective equipment (PPE) to staff and provide "just-in-time" training for staff participating in contaminated patient care?

5. Does your hospital consider the possibility of being a secondary terrorist target and take appropriate measures to protect the facility?

6. Does your hospital have a security plan to lock down the facility and control access and egress?

7. Does your hospital have a protocol or know the process for establishing contact with the alternate local EOC in the case of the primary local EOC being rendered nonfunctional by the blast?

8. Does your hospital's security plan include the preservation and securing of evidence, contaminated patient belongings, and specimens?

9. Does your hospital have a procedure to interface with local, state, and federal law enforcement agencies to interview patients, gather evidence, and investigate the incident?

10. Does your hospital prepare for the possibility that the perpetrator(s) is among the injured?

11. Does your hospital have a procedure/system to obtain current information from local officials about the RDD (e.g., plume direction, weather considerations, damage assessments, progress reports, etc.)?

12. Does your hospital have a communications plan that includes coordination with the local public health department and the local EOC/joint information center (JIC)?

13. Does your hospital have a triage process to separate contaminated victims from noncontaminated persons presenting for care that were not involved in the incident?

14. Does your hospital have procedures to manage radioactive shrapnel in traumatically injured and contaminated patients in surgery?

15. Does your hospital have procedures to manage arriving patients with blast injuries?

16. Does your hospital have a system and procedures to determine status of other area hospitals?

17. Does your hospital have a procedure to obtain specialized equipment and supplies?

18. Does your hospital have a procedure to establish a media conference area and provide regular briefings and updates, in collaboration with the JIC?

19. Does your hospital have criteria to prioritize business continuity and recovery activities?

20. Does your hospital have procedures to manage contaminated fatalities in conjunction with medical examiner and emergency management agency?

21. Does your hospital have a procedure to track patients, beds, personnel, and materiel?

22. Does your hospital have a facility decontamination plan and procedures?

23. Does your hospital have procedures to restore the facility and operations to normal?

24. Does your hospital have a plan to provide mental health support and stress management debriefings to staff, patients, and families?

RADIOLOGICAL ATTACK—RADIOLOGICAL DISPERSAL DEVICES

INCIDENT RESPONSE GUIDE

Mission: To provide care to radiologically contaminated and blast injuries after a terrorist attack with a radiological dispersal device that does not directly impact or contaminate the hospital.

Directions

☐ Read this entire response guide and review incident management team chart

☐ Use this response guide as a checklist to ensure all tasks are addressed and completed

Objectives

☐ Protect the facility, patients, and staff from contamination and injury

☐ Detect and monitor radiation levels

☐ Provide patient care and decontamination

☐ Communicate with the local emergency operations center (EOC) and emergency response partners

☐ Cooperate with and assist law enforcement with investigative activities

☐ Safely decontaminate the facility and restore normal operations

Immediate (Operational Period 0–2 Hours)

COMMAND

(Incident Commander):

    ☐ Appoint Command Staff, Section Chiefs, and Medical/Technical Specialist—Radiological

    ☐ Activate the emergency operations plan and the radiological decontamination plan

    ☐ Determine the radiological threat to the facility and the need for shelter-in-place

[Public Information Officer (PIO)]:

☐

    ☐ Establish a media staging area and prepare media briefings in collaboration with the joint information center and other area hospitals

(Liaison Officer):

    ☐ Establish contact with the alternate local EOC, other response partners, and area hospitals to determine incident details, community status, and estimates of casualties

    ☐ Contact appropriate authorities and experts for support and recommendations for radiological contamination

RADIOLOGICAL ATTACK—RADIOLOGICAL DISPERSAL DEVICES

INCIDENT RESPONSE GUIDE

COMMAND

(Safety Officer):

- ☐ Ensure activation of the radiological decontamination plan
- ☐ Ensure the safe and consistent use of appropriate personal protective equipment by staff

(Medical/Technical Specialist-Radiological):

- ☐ Assist in obtaining specific information regarding radiological agent such as antidotes, treatment, decontamination procedures, etc.

OPERATIONS

- ☐ Activate the radiological decontamination plan
- ☐ Secure the facility and establish access and egress routes and crowd control protocols
- ☐ Conduct a census of inpatients and clinic patients and prioritize for discharge or cancellation of appointment/procedures to accommodate the incoming surge of patients
- ☐ Activate the shelter-in-place plan, if necessary
- ☐ Establish and secure area(s) for collection of contaminated belongings and valuables

PLANNING

- ☐ Initiate patient, bed, personnel, and materiel tracking
- ☐ Establish operational periods and develop Incident Action Plan, in collaboration with the Incident Commander
- ☐ Initiate patient, bed, personnel, and materiel tracking
- ☐ Establish operational periods and develop incident objectives and the Incident Action Plan, in collaboration with the Incident Commander

LOGISTICS

- ☐ Ensure internal and external communications as well as IT/IS systems are operational
- ☐ Initiate staff radiation monitoring
- ☐ Anticipate an increased need for medical and surgical supplies, medications, and equipment and take action to obtain needed supplies
- ☐ Initiate staff call-in systems to increase hospital staffing

RADIOLOGICAL ATTACK—RADIOLOGICAL DISPERSAL DEVICES

INCIDENT RESPONSE GUIDE

Intermediate (Operational Period 2–12 Hours)

COMMAND

(Incident Commander):

- ☐ Review the overall impact of the ongoing incident on the facility with Command Staff and Section Chiefs
- ☐ Reevaluate the need to shelter-in-place
- ☐ Consider deploying a Liaison Officer to the alternate local EOC

[Public Information Officer (PIO)]:

- ☐ Establish a patient information center, coordinate with the Liaison Officer
- ☐ Establish a media center and conduct regular media briefings
- ☐ Coordinate messages with the joint information center

☐ (Liaison):

- ☐ Contact area hospitals and healthcare partners through local emergency management to assess their capabilities
- ☐ Maintain communication with the local EOC to relay hospital status and requests and obtain current situation status information

(Safety Officer):

- ☐ Continue to monitor and ensure proper use of personal protective equipment and decontamination procedures
- ☐ Conduct ongoing analysis of existing response practices for health and safety issues related to staff, patients, and facility, and implement corrective actions to address

(Medical/Technical Specialist-Radiological):

- ☐ Support Operations Section as needed; continue to provide expert input into Incident Action Planning process

OPERATIONS

☐
- ☐ Activate fatalities management plan and management of contaminated remains

PLANNING

☐
- ☐ Update and revise the incident objectives and the Incident Action Plan
- ☐ Continue patient, bed, personnel, and materiel tracking

RADIOLOGICAL ATTACK—RADIOLOGICAL DISPERSAL DEVICES

INCIDENT RESPONSE GUIDE

LOGISTICS

☐
- ☐ Continue employee monitoring for radiation and provide appropriate follow up
- ☐ Establish family care area, if needed
- ☐ Continue to inventory supplies, equipment, blood products, and medications; obtain additional supplies as needed
- ☐ Ensure safety of the facility and provide essential services
- ☐ Initiate staff call-in and provide additional staff to impacted areas

FINANCE

☐
- ☐ Track response expenses and expenditures
- ☐ Investigate staff or patient exposures or injuries and implement risk management/claims procedures

Extended (Operational Period Beyond 12 Hours)

COMMAND

(Incident Commander):

- ☐ Reassess incident objectives and Incident Action Plan, revise as indicated by the response priorities and mission

(PIO):

- ☐ Provide briefings and situation updates for staff, patients, visitors and families
- ☐ Continue to conduct regular media briefings in coordination with the JIC

☐
(Safety Officer):

- ☐ Continue to oversee safety measures and use of personal protective equipment for staff, patients, and visitors
- ☐ Monitor radiation exposures and decontamination operations

(Medical/Technical Specialist-Radiological):

- ☐ Continue to support Operations Section as needed; continue to provide expert input into Incident Action Planning process

RADIOLOGICAL ATTACK—RADIOLOGICAL DISPERSAL DEVICES

INCIDENT RESPONSE GUIDE

OPERATIONS

    ☐ Continue patient care and management activities

    ☐ Continue security measures and control of traffic and crowds

☐   ☐ Ensure enforcement of hospital policies and provide liaison with local, state, and federal law enforcement agencies when interviewing patients and collecting evidence

    ☐ Provide for facility decontamination

    ☐ Initiate return to normal activities of the hospital, as appropriate

---

PLANNING

☐   ☐ Continue patient, bed, materiel, and personnel tracking

    ☐ Update and revise the Incident Action Plan, in collaboration with the Incident Commander

---

FINANCE

☐   ☐ Continue to track response costs and expenditures and prepare regular reports for the Incident Commander

    ☐ Facilitate procurement of needed supplies, equipment, and contractors

---

Demobilization/System Recovery

COMMAND

(Incident Commander):

    ☐ Ensure demobilization and recovery is in progress

    ☐ Announce termination of event or "all clear" when appropriate

☐ (PIO):

    ☐ Conduct final media briefing including hospital status, appropriate patient information, and incident status, in coordination with the JIC

    ☐ Deactivate the patient information center

    ☐ Communicate final status to the JIC

RADIOLOGICAL ATTACK—RADIOLOGICAL DISPERSAL DEVICES

INCIDENT RESPONSE GUIDE

COMMAND

(Liaison Officer):

☐
- ☐ Communicate hospital status and demobilization to the local EOC, area hospitals and other local officials

(Safety Officer):

- ☐ Ensure safe return of hospital to normal operations
- ☐ Ensure facility decontamination

OPERATIONS

☐
- ☐ Return patient care and services to normal operations
- ☐ Ensure decontamination of facility
- ☐ Ensure proper disposal of contaminated waste and waste water
- ☐ Provide mental health support services for patients and their families

---

PLANNING

☐
- ☐ Write after-action report and improvement plan to include the following:
  - Summary of actions taken
  - Summary of the incident
  - Actions that went well
  - Area for improvement
  - Recommendations for future response actions
  - Recommendations for correction actions

LOGISTICS

☐
- ☐ Restock all hospital supplies, equipment, and medications to normal levels
- ☐ Initiate long term monitoring of employees exposed to radiation and/or participating in decontamination or patient care activities
- ☐ Assist in restoring hospital services to normal operations
- ☐ Provide mental health support and stress management services, as appropriate

---

RADIOLOGICAL ATTACK—RADIOLOGICAL DISPERSAL DEVICES

INCIDENT RESPONSE GUIDE

FINANCE

☐　　☐　Compile final response and recovery expenditure and expense reports and submit to the Incident Commander for approval and to distribution to appropriate authorities for reimbursement

---

Documents and Tools

☐　Hospital Emergency Preparedness Plan

☐　Disaster Plan Call List

☐　Hospital Damage Assessment Procedures

☐　Hospital Decontamination Plan

☐　HICS forms

RADIOLOGICAL ATTACK—
RADIOLOGICAL DISPERSAL DEVICES
INCIDENT MANAGEMENT TEAM CHART—**IMMEDIATE**

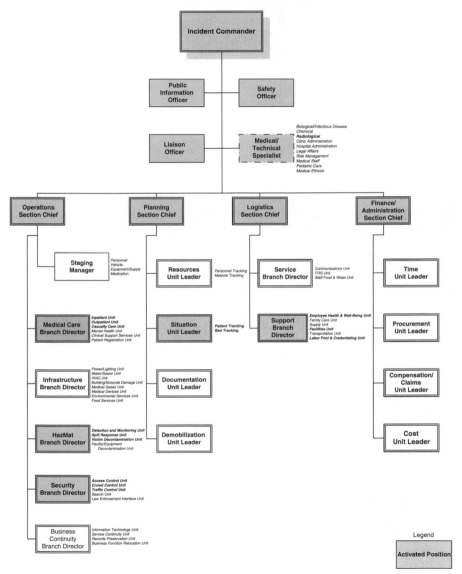

Incident Commander

Public Information Officer

Safety Officer

Liaison Officer

Medical/ Technical Specialist

Biological/Infectious Disease
Chemical
Radiological
Clinic Administration
Hospital Administration
Legal Affairs
Risk Management
Medical Staff
Pediatric Care
Medical Ethicist

Operations Section Chief

Planning Section Chief

Logistics Section Chief

Finance/ Administration Section Chief

Staging Manager
Personnel
Vehicle
Equipment/Supply
Medication

Resources Unit Leader
Personnel Tracking
Material Tracking

Service Branch Director
Communications Unit
IT/IS Unit
Staff Food & Water Unit

Time Unit Leader

Medical Care Branch Director
Inpatient Unit
Outpatient Unit
Casualty Care Unit
Mental Health Unit
Clinical Support Services Unit
Patient Registration Unit

Situation Unit Leader
Patient Tracking
Bed Tracking

Support Branch Director
Employee Health & Well-Being Unit
Family Care Unit
Supply Unit
Facilities Unit
Transportation Unit
Labor Pool & Credentialing Unit

Procurement Unit Leader

Infrastructure Branch Director
Power/Lighting Unit
Water/Sewer Unit
HVAC Unit
Building/Grounds Damage Unit
Medical Gases Unit
Medical Devices Unit
Environmental Services Unit
Food Services Unit

Documentation Unit Leader

Compensation/ Claims Unit Leader

HazMat Branch Director
Detection and Monitoring Unit
Spill Response Unit
Victim Decontamination Unit
Facility/Equipment
   Decontamination Unit

Demobilization Unit Leader

Cost Unit Leader

Security Branch Director
Access Control Unit
Crowd Control Unit
Traffic Control Unit
Search Unit
Law Enforcement Interface Unit

Business Continuity Branch Director
Information Technology Unit
Service Continuity Unit
Records Preservation Unit
Business Function Relocation Unit

Legend

Activated Position

RADIOLOGICAL ATTACK—
RADIOLOGICAL DISPERSAL DEVICES
INCIDENT MANAGEMENT TEAM CHART—**INTERMEDIATE**

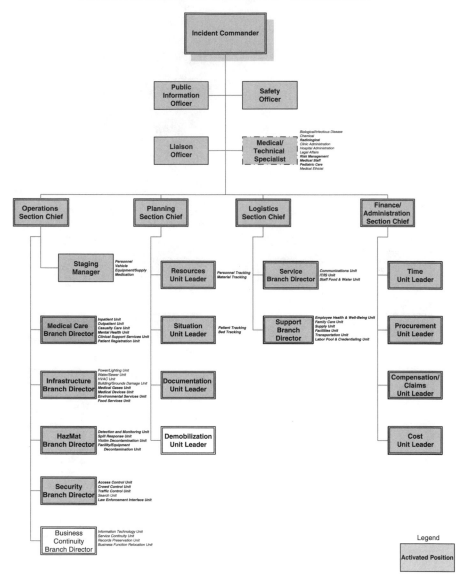

RADIOLOGICAL ATTACK—
RADIOLOGICAL DISPERSAL DEVICES

INCIDENT MANAGEMENT TEAM CHART—**EXTENDED**

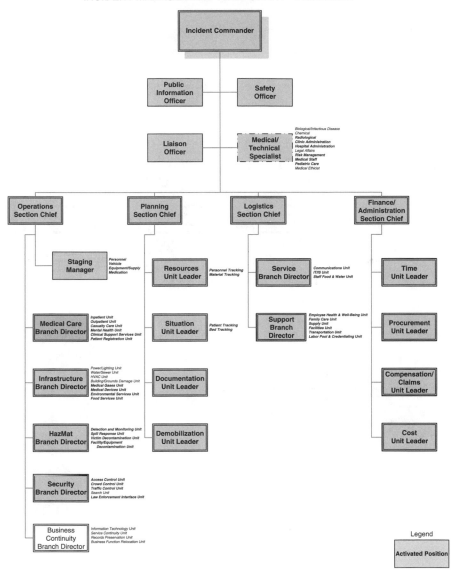

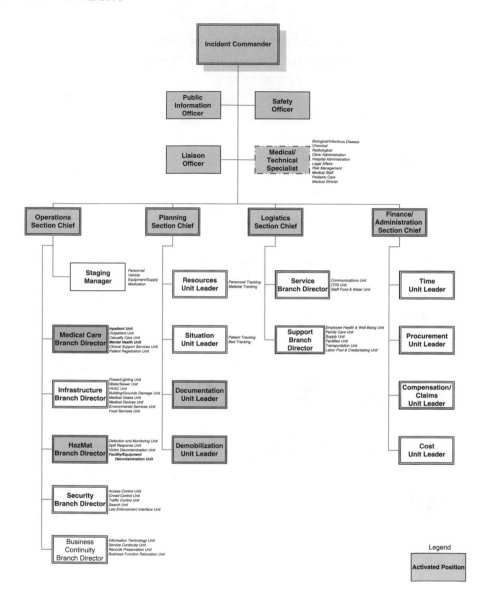

APPENDIX E

FEDERAL AGENCIES GOVERNING THE IMMEDIATE RESPONSE TO A RADIOLOGICAL EVENT

Source: The Nuclear/Radiological Incident Annex (NRIA) to the National Response Framework (NRF)

E.1 INTRODUCTION

E.1.1 Purpose

The Nuclear/Radiological Incident Annex (NRIA) to the National Response Framework (NRF) describes the policies, situations, concepts of operations, and responsibilities of the federal departments and agencies that govern the immediate response and short-term recovery activities for incidents involving release of radioactive materials to address the consequences of the event. These incidents may occur on federal-owned or -licensed facilities, privately owned property, urban centers, or other areas and may vary in severity from the small to the catastrophic. The incidents may result from inadvertent or deliberate acts. The NRIA applies to incidents where the nature and scope of the incident requires a federal response to supplement the state, tribal, or local incident response.

Radiation Safety: Protection and Management for Homeland Security and Emergency Response. By L. A. Burchfield
Copyright © 2009 John Wiley & Sons, Inc.

The purpose of this annex is as follows:

- Define the roles and responsibilities of federal agencies in responding to the unique characteristics of different categories of nuclear/radiological incidents
- Discuss the specific authorities, capabilities, and assets the federal government has for responding to nuclear/radiological incidents that are not otherwise described in the NRF
- Discuss the integration of the concept of operations with other elements of the NRF, which includes the unique organization, notification, and activation processes and the specialized incident-related actions
- Provide guidelines for notification, coordination, and leadership of federal activities

Because potential incidents and impacted entities fall into several categories this annex identifies different federal agencies as "coordinating agencies," and "cooperating agencies," and it examines associated strategic concepts of operations based on the authorities, responsibilities, and capabilities of those departments or agencies. In addition, this annex describes how other federal departments and agencies support the Department of Homeland Security (DHS) when DHS leads a large-scale, multiagency, federal response.

E.1.2 Scope

This annex applies to two categories of nuclear and radiological incidents: (1) inadvertent or otherwise accidental releases and (2) releases related to deliberate acts. These incidents may also include the potential release of radioactive material that poses an actual or perceived hazard to public health, safety, national security, and/or the environment. The category covering inadvertent releases includes two categories of nuclear facilities (commercial or weapons production facilities), lost radioactive material sources, transportation accidents that involve nuclear/radioactive material, domestic nuclear weapons accidents, and foreign accidents that involve nuclear or radioactive material that impact the United States or its territories, possessions, or territorial waters. The second category includes, but is not limited to, response to the effects of deliberate attacks perpetrated with radiological dispersal devices (RDDs), nuclear weapons, or improvised nuclear devices (INDs).

This annex applies whenever a federal response is undertaken unilaterally pursuant to federal authorities, or when an incident exceeds or is anticipated to exceed state, tribal, or local resources. The level of federal response to a specific incident is based on numerous factors, which include the ability of state, tribal, and local officials to respond; the type, amount, and custody of (or authority over) radioactive material involved; the extent of the impact or potential impact on the public and environment; and the size of the affected area.

If any agency or government entity becomes aware of an overt threat or act involving nuclear/radiological material/device or indications the event is not inadvertent or otherwise accidental, the Department of Justice (DOJ) should be notified through the Federal Bureau of Investigation (FBI). The Attorney General has lead responsibility for criminal investigations of terrorist acts or terrorist threats by individuals or groups inside the United States, or directed at United States citizens or institutions abroad, where such acts are within the federal criminal jurisdiction of the United States. Generally acting through the FBI, the Attorney General, in cooperation with other federal departments and agencies engaged in activities to protect our national security, shall also coordinate the activities of the other members of the law enforcement community to detect, prevent, preempt, and disrupt terrorist attacks against the United States. For investigations that pertain to nuclear/radiological incidents, the coordinating agencies and cooperating agencies perform the functions delineated in this annex and provide technical support and assistance to the FBI in the performance of its law enforcement and criminal investigative mission. More details regarding the FBI response are outlined in the Terrorism Incident Law Enforcement and Investigation Annex.

In situations that result from a deliberate act, NRIA response actions will be coordinated with the NRF and the Terrorism Incident Law Enforcement and Investigation Annex and the Catastrophic Incident Annex, as appropriate.

E.1.3 Policies

Authorities applicable to this annex include Homeland Security Presidential Directive (HSPD) 5 ("Management of Domestic Incidents"), the National Strategy to Combat Weapons of Mass Destruction, the Homeland Security Act of 2002, the Post-Katrina Emergency Management Reform Act of 2006 (PKEMRA), and the National Strategy for Homeland Security.

The coordinating agencies may take appropriate independent emergency actions within the limits of their own statutory authority to protect the public, mitigate immediate hazards, and gather information concerning the emergency to avoid delay. Key authorities used by the coordinating agencies in carrying out their responsibilities are described in the bullets below. Some of these authorities apply to multiple coordinating agencies.

- **Comprehensive Environmental Response, Compensation, and Liability Act (CERCLA)**—CERCLA gives the federal government the authority to respond to releases or threatened releases of hazardous substances (including radionuclides) that may endanger public health or the environment.[1] CERCLA also gives the federal government the authority to compel responsible parties to respond to releases of hazardous substances. CERCLA is implemented through the National Oil and Hazardous Substances Pollution Contingency Plan (NCP), a regulation found in 40 Code of Federal Regulation (CFR) Part 300. At the on-scene level, this response authority is implemented by federal On-Scene Coordinators (OSCs). OSCs may assist state and local governments in responding to releases but have the authority to direct the response when needed to ensure protection of public health and the environment. Typical response actions include, but are not limited to, air monitoring, assessment of the extent of the contamination, stabilization of the release, decontamination, waste treatment, storage, and disposal. Four federal agencies have OSC authority for hazardous substance emergencies: the Environmental Protection Agency (EPA), DHS/U.S. Coast Guard (USCG), the Department of Defense (DOD), and the Department of Energy (DOE).

- **Atomic Energy Act (AEA) of 1954 (as amended)**—The AEA provides DOD and DOE responsibilities for protection of certain nuclear materials, facilities, information, and nuclear weapons under their control. The AEA (42 U.S.C. §§ 2011–2297 (2003)) and the Energy Reorganization Act of 1974 (5 U.S.C. §§ 5313–5316, 42 U.S.C. §§ 5801–5891 (2002)) provide the statutory authority for both DOE and the Nuclear Regulatory Commission (NRC), and the foundation for NRC regulation of the nation's civilian use of by-product, source, and special nuclear materials to ensure adequate protection of public health and safety, to promote the common defense and security, and to protect the environment. For incidents that involve NRC- or Agreement State-regulated facilities, activities, or material, the NRC has the authority to perform an independent assessment of the safety of the facility or material; evaluate licensee protective action recommendations; perform oversight of the licensee (monitoring, advising, assisting, and/or directing); and report information, as appropriate, to media and public entities. The AEA also charges the EPA with additional responsibilities regarding radiation matters that directly or indirectly affect public health.

- **Executive Order 12656 of November 18, 1988**—This executive order directs the Secretary of Energy to "manage all emergency planning

---

[1]The definition of "release" under CERCLA excludes releases of source, by-product, or special nuclear material from a nuclear incident at certain facilities licensed by the Nuclear Regulatory Commission.

and response activities pertaining to Department of Energy nuclear facilities."

- **Title 50, U.S. Code, War and National Defense**—Title 50, U.S.C. § 797 makes it a crime willfully to violate a regulation or order promulgated by the Secretary of Defense, or by a military commander designated by the Secretary of Defense, for the protection or security of military equipment or other property or places subject to the jurisdiction, administration, or custody of DOD. As it applies to nuclear/radiological accidents or incidents, this statute provides a military commander the authority to establish a temporary National Defense Area (NDA) around an accident/incident site to protect nuclear weapons and materials in DOD custody. This statute is executed within the Department by DOD Instruction 5200.08, "Security of DOD Installations and Resources." DODI 5200.08 is the natural, legal extension of statutory authority found in 50 U.S.C. § 797.

- **Public Health Service Act (PHSA)**—The PHSA directs the EPA to support state and local authorities in their preparedness and response activities regarding public health emergencies. This support could include providing training, technical advice, and direct assistance. The PHSA created the Environmental Health Service, whose mission included radiological health. This mission was carried out by the Bureau of Radiological Health (BRH).

The definition of "release" under CERCLA excludes releases of source, by-product, or special nuclear material from a nuclear incident at certain facilities licensed by the Nuclear Regulatory Commission. Reorganization Plan Number 3 of 1970, which created the EPA, transferred certain radiological health functions of the BRH to the EPA.

The NRF, like its predecessor, the National Response Plan (NRP), supersedes the Federal Radiological Emergency Response Plan (FRERP) dated May 1, 1996.

DHS/Federal Emergency Management Agency (FEMA) is responsible for maintaining and updating this annex. DHS/FEMA accomplishes this responsibility through the Federal Radiological Preparedness Coordinating Committee (FRPCC).

When DHS initiates the response mechanisms of the NRF, including the emergency support functions (ESFs), appropriate NRF Support Annexes, and this annex, existing interagency plans that address nuclear/radiological incident management [e.g., the National Oil and Hazardous Substances Pollution Contingency Plan (NCP)] are incorporated as supporting plans and/or operational supplements to the NRF.

For incidents not led by DHS, other federal agency response plans provide the primary federal response protocols. In these cases, the federal agency that is coordinating the federal response may use the procedures outlined in the NRF and in appropriate NRF annexes to coordinate the delivery of federal resources to state, tribal, and local governments, and to coordinate assistance among federal agencies for incidents requiring federal coordination.

Certain federal agencies are authorized to respond directly to specific nuclear/radiological incidents. Nothing in this annex alters or impedes the ability of federal departments and agencies to carry out their specific authorities and to perform their responsibilities under law. This annex does not create any new authorities and does not change any existing ones.

Federal response actions will be carried out commensurate with the appropriate health and safety laws and guidelines. For example, if the area is contaminated by radioactive material, and appropriate personal protective equipment and capabilities are not available, response actions may be delayed until the material has dissipated to a safe level for emergency response personnel or until appropriate personal protective equipment and capabilities arrive.

The federal government has established protective action guides (PAGs) for radiological incidents. Specific PAGs have also been established for RDD/INDs.

Federal coordination centers and agency teams provide their own logistical support consistent with agreed-upon interagency execution plans. State, tribal, and local governments are encouraged to coordinate their efforts with the federal effort, but they maintain their own logistical support, which is consistent with applicable authorities and requirements.

The federal response to any nuclear/radiological incident shall be coordinated with the state, tribal, and local government or the federal agencies that have jurisdiction over the area affected by the incident. Response to nuclear/radiological incidents affecting land owned by the federal government is coordinated with the agency responsible for managing that land to ensure that incident management activities are consistent with federal statutes that govern use and occupancy. In the case of tribal lands, tribal governments have a special relationship with the U.S. Government, and federal, state, and local governments may have limited or no authority on specific tribal reservations. More guidance is provided in the Tribal Relations Support Annex.

E.1.4 Headquarters Planning and Preparedness

Under existing regulations, the FRPCC provides a national-level forum for the development and coordination of radiological planning and preparedness policies and procedures. It also provides policy guidance for federal radiological incident management activities in support of state, tribal, and local government radiological emergency planning and preparedness activities. The FRPCC is an interagency body that consists of the coordinating and cooperating agencies discussed in this annex, chaired by DHS/FEMA.

The FRPCC also coordinates research-study efforts of its member agencies related to state, tribal, and local government radiological emergency preparedness to ensure minimum duplication and maximum benefits to state and local governments. The FRPCC coordinates planning and validating requirements of each agency, reviewing integration requirements and incorporating agency-specific plans, procedures, and equipment into the response system.

As part of their preparedness for nuclear/radiological emergencies, federal agencies participate in exercises to test and evaluate response plans. Regional Planning and Preparedness Coordinating agencies may have regional offices or field structures that provide a forum for information sharing, consultation, and coordination of federal agency regional awareness, prevention, preparedness, response, and recovery activities for radiological incidents. These regional offices may also assist in providing technical assistance to State and local governments and evaluating radiological plans and exercises.

Regional Assistance Committees (RACs) in the DHS/FEMA regions serve as the primary coordinating structures at the federal regional level. RAC membership mirrors that of the FRPCC, and RACs are chaired by a DHS/FEMA regional representative. Additionally, states send representatives to RAC meetings and participate in regional exercise and training activities. The RACs provide a forum for information sharing, consultation, and coordination of federal regional awareness, prevention, preparedness, response, and recovery activities. The RACs also assist in providing technical assistance to state and local governments in evaluating radiological plans and exercises.

E.2 SITUATION

A nuclear/radiological incident may result from a deliberate act, an accident, or general mismanagement, and may center around different materials or industrial practices, which include the following:

- Commercial nuclear facilities
- Federal nuclear weapons facilities
- Radioactive material sources, industrial uses, or technologically enhanced, naturally occurring radioactive material
- Transportation incidents that involve nuclear/radioactive material
- Domestic nuclear weapons accidents

- Foreign incidents involving nuclear or radioactive materials
- Terrorism involving facilities or nuclear/radiological materials, including the use of RDDs or INDs

The most common nuclear/radiological incidents have to do with the loss, theft, or mismanagement of relatively small radioactive material sources, or technologically enhanced, naturally occurring radioactive material, where some exposure of individuals or dispersal into the environment occurs. These incidents are handled at the local level with occasional federal assistance. Generally, greater regulatory control, safeguards, and security accompany larger quantities of radioactive materials, which pose a greater potential threat to human health and the environment.

Virtually any facility or industrial practice (including transportation of materials) may be vulnerable to a deliberate act, such as terrorism, or an accident of some sort that could release radioactive material, which includes a fire. Major fixed facilities, such as federal nuclear weapons facilities, commercial nuclear fuel cycle facilities (uranium enrichment, fuel fabrication, power reactors, and disposal), and some nonfuel cycle industries (such as radiation source and radiopharmaceutical manufacturers) pose a risk of accidents and could also be breached in a deliberate act, such as terrorism.

A radiological dispersal device is any device used to spread radioactive material into the environment with malicious intent. The harm caused by an RDD is principally contamination, and denial of use of the contaminated area, perhaps for many years. The costs to the nation associated with an effective RDD could be very significant. Of greatest concern to U.S. security is the potential for a terrorist attack using a nuclear weapon. A nuclear device could originate directly from a nuclear state, be modified from preexisting weapons components, or be fashioned by terrorists from the basic fissile nuclear materials (uranium-235 or plutonium-239). Even a small nuclear detonation in an urban area could result in over 100,000 fatalities (and many more injured), massive infrastructure damage, and thousands of square kilometers of contaminated land.

E.3 PLANNING ASSUMPTIONS

Radiological incidents may not be immediately recognized as such until the radioactive material is detected or the health effects of radiation exposure are manifested in the population and identified by the public health community.

An act of nuclear or radiological terrorism, particularly an act directed against a large population center within the United States, can have major consequences that can overwhelm the capabilities of many local, tribal, and/or state governments to respond, and may seriously challenge existing federal response capabilities.

An act or threat of nuclear or radiological terrorism will trigger concurrent activation of the Terrorism Law Enforcement and Investigation Annex.

A nuclear or radiological incident may require concurrent implementation of the NCP to address radiological, as well as chemical or biological, releases into the environment.

An incident that involves the potential release of radioactivity may require implementation of protective measures, such as evacuation and shelter-in-place. State, tribal, and local governments have primary responsibility for implementing protective measures for the public.

An expeditious federal response is required to mitigate the consequences of a nuclear/radiological incident. The federal government response to nuclear or radiological terrorist threats/incidents includes, but is not limited to, the following assumptions:

- The response to a radiological threat or actual incident requires an integrated federal government response.
- In the case of a nuclear terrorist attack, the plume may be dispersed over a large area over time, which requires response operations to be conducted over a multijurisdictional and/or multistate region.
- A terrorist attack may involve multiple incidents, and each location may require an incident response and a crime scene investigation simultaneously.

E.4 RESPONSIBILITIES

E.4.1 General

Incidents will be managed at the lowest possible level; as incidents change in size, scope, and complexity, the response will adapt to meet requirements, as described in the NRF. In accordance with HSPD-5, "the Secretary of Homeland Security is the principal federal official for domestic incident management. The Secretary is responsible for coordinating federal operations within the United States to prepare for, respond to, and recover from terrorist attacks, major disasters, and other emergencies. The Secretary shall coordinate the federal government's resources utilized in response to or recovery from terrorist attacks, major disasters, or other emergencies. . . ." Domestic incident management includes preventing, preparing for, responding to, and recovering from terrorist attacks (except for those law enforcement coordination activities

TABLE E.1 Coordinating Agencies for Nuclear/Radiological Incidents

Nuclear/Radiological Facilities or Materials Involved in Incident	Coordinating Agency
Nuclear facilities:	
(1) Owned or operated by DOD or DOE	(1) DOD or DOE
(2) Licensed by NRC or Agreement State	(2) NRC
(3) Not licensed, owned, or operated by a federal agency or an Agreement State, or currently or formerly licensed facilities for which the owner/operator is not financially viable or is otherwise unable to respond	(3) EPA
Radioactive materials being transported:	
(1) Materials shipped by or for DOD or DOE[2]	(1) DOD or DOE
(2) Shipment of NRC or Agreement State-licensed materials	(2) NRC
(3) Shipment of materials in certain areas of the coastal zone that are not licensed or owned by a federal agency or Agreement State (see DHS/USCG list of responsibilities for further explanation of "certain areas")	(3) DHS/USCG
(4) All others	(4) EPA
Radioactive materials in space vehicles impacting within the United States:	
(1) Managed by NASA or DOD	(1) NASA or DOD
(2) Not managed by DOD or NASA and impacting certain areas of the coastal zone	(2) DHS/USCG
(3) All others	(3) EPA
Foreign, unknown, or unlicensed material:[3]	
(1) Incidents involving inadvertent import of radioactive materials	(1) DHS/CBP
(2) Incidents involving foreign or unknown sources of radioactive material in certain areas of the coastal zone	(2) DHS/USCG
(3) All others	(3) EPA

(Continued)

[2]The coordinating agency is either DOD or DOE, depending on which of these agencies has custody of the material at the time of the incident.
[3]The DHS Domestic Nuclear Detection Office (DNDO) coordinates the adjudication of unresolved radiation detection alarms (see Table E.5 for additional information).

TABLE E.1   *Continued*

Nuclear/Radiological Facilities or Materials Involved in Incident	Coordinating Agency
Nuclear weapons	DOD or DOE (based on custody at time of incident)
All deliberate attacks involving nuclear/radiological facilities or materials, including RDDs or INDs[4,5]	DHS

Note: When exercising domestic incident management responsibilities, the Secretary of Homeland Security is supported by other coordinating agencies and cooperating agencies. For incidents wherein the Secretary is not fulfilling domestic incident management responsibilities, the coordinating agency will be the responsible agency for domestic incident management as defined by their authorities.

assigned to the Attorney General and generally delegated to the Director of the FBI set forth in HSPD-5, paragraph 8). When exercising this role, the Secretary is supported by other coordinating agencies and cooperating agencies. For incidents wherein the Secretary is not fulfilling domestic incident management responsibilities, the coordinating agency will be the responsible agency for domestic incident management as defined by their authorities. Such incidents include, but are not limited to, loss of radiography sources, discovery of orphan radiological sources, and incidents/emergencies at nuclear facilities below the classification of General Emergency, as defined by the cognizant coordinating agency.

- For this annex, coordinating agencies provide the leadership, expertise, and authorities to implement critical and specific nuclear/radiological aspects of the response, and facilitate nuclear/radiological aspects of the response in accordance with those authorities and capabilities. The coordinating agencies are those federal agencies that own, have custody of, authorize, regulate, or are otherwise assigned responsibility for the nuclear/radioactive material, facility, or activity involved in the incident. These federal agencies have nuclear/radiological authorities, technical expertise, and/or assets for responding to the unique characteristics of nuclear/radiological incidents that are not otherwise described in the NRF. Coordinating agencies are listed in Table E.1. The specific role

[4]For deliberate attacks, DHS assumes its domestic incident management responsibilities under HSPD-5, paragraph 4, and it is also the coordinating agency for implementing the activities in this annex with respect to deliberate attacks.
[5]For deliberate attacks, DOJ assumes those law enforcement coordination activities under HSPD-5, paragraph 8.

of each coordinating agency will be determined by the scope of their particular authorities over relevant aspects of the incident, as described in more detail in this annex.

- Cooperating agencies include other federal agencies that provide additional technical and resource support specific to nuclear/radiological incidents to DHS and the coordinating agencies. The capabilities provided by cooperating agencies are described in Table E.5 at the end of this annex.
- Other federal agencies may also provide support to DHS and the coordinating agency in accordance with the ESF and Support Annexes.

E.4.2   Coordinating Agencies

For nuclear/radiological incidents, the coordinating agencies include the following Federal agencies:

- DOD or DOE as appropriate, for incidents that involve nuclear/radiological materials or facilities owned or operated by DOD or DOE.
- DOD or DOE, as appropriate, for incidents that involve a nuclear weapon, special nuclear material, and/or classified components under DOD or DOE custody.
- National Aeronautics and Space Administration (NASA) for nuclear material under NASA custody.
- The NRC, for incidents that involve materials or facilities licensed by the NRC or Agreement States.
- DHS, generally through Customs and Border Protection (CBP), for incidents that involve the inadvertent import of radioactive materials as well as any other incidents where radioactive material is detected at borders.
- EPA or DHS/USCG, as appropriate, for environmental response and cleanup for incidents not otherwise covered above.
- DHS for all deliberate attacks involving nuclear/radiological facilities or materials, including RDDs and INDs.

Table E.1 provides an overview of the coordinating agencies and the types of nuclear/radiological incidents in which they will be involved. The specific responsibilities of coordinating agencies are further described in Table E.2.

Table E.2 below presents the specific responsibilities of each coordinating agency, as specified by statutory authorities or other mandating doctrine.

TABLE E.2   Coordinating Agency-Specific Key Responsibilities for
a Nuclear/Radiological Incident

Agency	Description
Department of Defense	As indicated in Table E.1, the DOD is the coordinating agency for federal actions related to radiological incidents that involve nuclear weapons in DOD custody; DOD facilities, including U.S. nuclear-powered ships; or material otherwise under DOD jurisdiction (e.g., transportation of material shipped by or for DOD). Under CERCLA, Executive Order 12580, and the NCP, the DOD is responsible for hazardous substance responses to releases on or from DOD facilities or vessels under the jurisdiction, custody, or control of DOD, including transportation-related incidents. For responses under these circumstances, DOD provides a federal OSC responsible for taking all CERCLA response actions, which includes on-site and off-site response actions (40 CFR 300.120(c) and 40 CFR 300.175(b)(4)). For incidents where the incident is on, or where the sole source of the nuclear/radiological release is from, any facility or vessel under DOD jurisdiction, custody, or control, the DOD is responsible for: • Mitigating the consequences of an incident. • Providing notification and appropriate protective action recommendations to State, tribal, and/or local government officials. • Minimizing the radiological hazard to the public. For radiological incidents involving a nuclear weapon, special nuclear material, and/or classified components that are in DOD custody, the DOD may establish a National Defense Area. The DOD will coordinate with state and local officials to ensure appropriate public health and safety actions are taken outside the NDA. The DOD will lead the overall response to safeguard national security information and/or restricted data, or equipment and material. The DOD may also include lands normally not under DOD control as part of the established NDA for the duration of the incident. The DOD coordinates the federal response for incidents involving the release of nuclear/radioactive materials from DOD space vehicles or joint space vehicles with significant DOD involvement. A joint venture is an activity in which the U.S. Government has provided extensive design/financial input; has provided and maintains ownership of instruments, spacecraft, or the launch vehicle; or is intimately involved in mission operations. A joint venture with a foreign nation is not created by simply selling or

(Continued)

TABLE E.2 *Continued*

Agency	Description

supplying material to a foreign country for use in its spacecraft.

In the event that the DHS assumes overall management of the federal response under HSPD-5 to an accidental or inadvertent incident involving DOD facilities or materials, the DOD will support the DHS under the NRF and the National Incident Management System (NIMS), including acting as the coordinating agency for this annex. The DOD will manage the response within the boundaries of the DOD facility or NDA.

Department of Energy

As indicated in Table E.1, the DOE is the coordinating agency for the federal response to a nuclear/radiological release at a DOE facility or involving DOE materials (e.g., during the use, storage, and shipment of a variety of radioactive materials; the shipment of spent reactor fuel; the production, assembly, and shipment of nuclear weapons and special nuclear materials; the production and shipment of radioactive sources for space ventures; and the storage and shipment of radioactive and mixed waste).

Under CERCLA, Executive Order 12580, and the NCP, the DOE is responsible for hazardous substance responses to releases on or from DOE facilities or vessels under the jurisdiction, custody, or control of the DOE, including transportation-related incidents. For responses under these circumstances, the DOE provides a federal OSC responsible for taking all CERCLA response actions, which includes on-site and off-site response actions (40 CFR 300.120(c) and 40 CFR 300.175(b)(5)).

For incidents at nuclear/radiological facilities that it owns or operates, or incidents involving transportation of DOE nuclear/radiological materials, the DOE is responsible for:

- Mitigating the consequences of an incident
- Providing notification and appropriate protective action recommendations to State, tribal, and/or local government officials
- Minimizing the radiological hazard to the public

For radiological incidents that involve a nuclear weapon, special nuclear material, and/or classified components that are in DOE custody, the DOE may establish a National Security Area (NSA). The DOE will coordinate with state and local officials to ensure appropriate public health and safety actions are taken outside the NSA. The DOE will lead the overall response to safeguard national security information and/or restricted data, or equipment and material. The DOE may also include lands normally not

(Continued)

TABLE E.2   *Continued*

Agency	Description
	under DOE control as part of the established NSA for the duration of the incident.
	The DOE Accident Response Group (ARG) teams will deploy to mitigate the consequences of a nuclear weapon accident in conjunction with specialized assets from DOD, regardless of whether DOE or DOD has custody of the weapon or special nuclear material.
	In the event that DHS assumes overall management of the federal response under HSPD-5 to an accidental or inadvertent incident involving DOE facilities or materials, the DOE will support DHS under the NRF and NIMS, including acting as the coordinating agency for this annex. The DOE will manage the response within the boundaries of the DOE facility or NSA.
Department of Homeland Security	The Secretary of Homeland Security is the principal federal official for domestic incident management. Domestic incident management includes preventing, preparing for, responding to, and recovering from terrorist attacks (except for those law enforcement coordination activities assigned to the Attorney General and generally delegated to the Director of the FBI), major disasters, or other emergencies.
	For deliberate attacks, the DHS assumes its domestic incident management responsibilities under HSPD-5, paragraph 4, and is also the coordinating agency for implementing the activities in this annex with respect to deliberate attacks.
	Under the Homeland Security Act, the DHS has control of the Nuclear Incident Response Team (NIRT).
	DHS/CBP coordinates the federal response for incidents involving the inadvertent import of radioactive material.
	For incidents at the border, DHS/CBP maintains radiation detection equipment and nonintrusive inspection technology at ports of entry and border patrol checkpoints to detect the presence of radiological substances transported by persons, cargo, mail, or conveyance arriving from foreign countries.
	DHS/U.S. Coast Guard.
	As indicated in Table E.1, DHS/USCG is the coordinating agency for the federal response to incidents involving the release of nuclear/radioactive materials that occur in certain areas of the coastal zone, including the following:
	• Release from transportation incidents involving the release of nuclear/radioactive materials that are not licensed or owned by a federal agency or Agreement State
	• Incidents involving space vehicles not managed by DOD or NASA that impact certain areas of the coastal zone

(Continued)

TABLE E.2 *Continued*

Agency	Description

- Incidents involving foreign or unknown sources of radioactive material
- "Certain areas" of the coastal zone, for the purposes of this document, means the following areas of the coastal zone ("coastal zone" as defined by the NCP):
  - Vessels, as defined in 33 CFR 160
  - Areas seaward of the shoreline to the outer edge of the Economic Exclusion Zone

Within the boundaries of the following waterfront facilities subject to the jurisdiction of DHS/USCG: those regulated by 33 CFR 126 (Dangerous cargo handling), 127 (LPG/LNG), 128 (Passenger terminals), 140 (Outer continental shelf activities), 154–156 (Waterfront portions of oil and hazmat bulk transfer facilities—delineated as per the NCP), 105 (Maritime security—facilities).

For incidents that have cross-boundary impacts, there will be only one OSC during the course of a response incident, and the agencies involved should reference the NCP [40 CFR 300.140(b)] to determine which agency will assume the lead. DHS/USCG will give prime consideration to the area vulnerable to the greatest threat in determining whether to transition to another coordinating agency.

DHS/USCG coordinates agency response for these incidents during the prevention and emergency response phase, and it transfers responsibility for later response phases to the appropriate agency.

Environmental Protection Agency

As indicated in Table E.1, the EPA is the coordinating agency for the federal environmental response to incidents that occur at facilities not licensed, owned, or operated by a federal agency or an Agreement State, or currently or formerly licensed facilities for which the owner/operator is not financially viable or otherwise cannot respond. The EPA is also the coordinating agency for the federal environmental response to incidents that involve the release of nuclear/radioactive materials that occur in the inland zone and in areas of the coastal zone not addressed by DHS/USCG, including the following:

- Transportation incidents involving the release of nuclear/radioactive materials that are not licensed or owned by a federal agency or Agreement State
- Incidents involving space vehicles not managed by DOD or NASA or addressed by DHS/USCG
- Incidents involving foreign, unknown, or unlicensed radiological sources that have actual, potential, or

(Continued)

TABLE E.2   *Continued*

Agency	Description
	perceived radiological consequences in the United States or its territories, possessions, or territorial waters, and that are not addressed by DHS/CBP or DHS/USCG
	When acting as the coordinating agency, the EPA coordinates the federal environmental response. For a DHS-led federal response, the EPA will generally be providing that response coordination support to the DHS through this annex and ESF #10—Oil and Hazardous Materials Response. For an EPA-led federal response, the EPA will generally be responding under the NCP (which is an operational supplement to the NRF). For some incidents, the EPA may also be relying on its Public Health Service Act authorities.
National Aeronautics and Space Administration	As indicated in Table E.1, NASA is the coordinating agency for the federal response to incidents involving the release of nuclear/radioactive materials from NASA space vehicles or joint space vehicles with significant NASA involvement. For radiological incidents involving nuclear material in NASA custody, NASA may establish an NSA, and will coordinate with state and local officials to ensure appropriate public health and safety actions are taken outside the NSA. In the event that the DHS assumes overall management of the federal response under HSPD-5 to an accidental or inadvertent incident involving NASA space vehicles, NASA will support the DHS under the NRF and NIMS, including acting as the coordinating agency for this annex. NASA will manage the response within the boundaries of the NSA.
Nuclear Regulatory Commission	As indicated in Table E.1, the NRC is the coordinating agency for incidents at or caused by a facility or an activity that is licensed by the NRC or an Agreement State. These facilities include, but are not limited to, commercial nuclear power plants, fuel cycle facilities, DOE-owned gaseous diffusion facilities operating under NRC regulatory oversight, independent spent fuel storage installations, radiopharmaceutical manufacturers, and research reactors.
	The NRC licensee primarily is responsible for taking action to mitigate the consequences of an incident and providing appropriate protective action recommendations to state, local, and/or tribal government officials. The NRC does the following:
	• Performs an independent assessment of the incident and potential off-site consequences and, as appropriate, provides recommendations concerning any protective measures

(Continued)

TABLE E.2 *Continued*

Agency	Description
	• Performs oversight of the licensee, to include monitoring, evaluation of protective action recommendations, advice, assistance, and, as appropriate, direction
	• Dispatches, if appropriate, an NRC site team of technical experts to the licensee's facility
	Under certain extraordinary situations that involve public health/safety or national defense/security, the NRC may order the transfer of special nuclear materials and/or the operation of certain facilities regulated by the NRC.
	The NRC closely coordinates its actions with state and local government officials during an incident by providing advice, guidance, and support as needed.
	In the event that the DHS assumes overall management of the federal response under HSPD-5 to an accidental or inadvertent incident involving an NRC-regulated facility, the NRC will support the DHS under the NRF and NIMS, including acting as the coordinating agency for this annex.

E.5 KEY FEDERAL RADIOLOGICAL RESOURCES/ASSETS

In carrying out their responsibilities, the DHS and coordinating agencies may request specialized assets for nuclear/radiological response. Some assets are provided by individual cooperating agencies (through ESF activations or their own authorities), whereas others may be interagency. Key specialized federal nuclear/radiological assets and teams are described below, whereas the procedures for activating these resources are described in the Concept of Operations section of this annex.

- Federal Radiological Monitoring and Assessment Center (FRMAC)—The FRMAC is responsible for coordinating all environmental radiological monitoring, sampling, and assessment activities for the response. The FRMAC is a DOE-led interagency asset that is available on request to respond to nuclear/radiological incidents. DOE leads the FRMAC for the initial response, then transitions FRMAC leadership to EPA for site cleanup. The FRMAC is established at or near the incident location in coordination with DHS, the coordinating agency, other federal agencies, and state, tribal, and local authorities.

A FRMAC normally includes representation from the DOE, the EPA, the Department of Commerce, the DHS National Communications System, the

U.S. Army Corps of Engineers (USACE), and other federal agencies as needed. Regardless of who is designated as the coordinating agency, when the FRMAC is activated, the DOE, through the FRMAC or DOE Consequence Management Home Team (CMHT), coordinates all federal environmental and agricultural radiological monitoring and assessment activities for the initial phases of the response. When the FRMAC is transferred to the EPA, the EPA assumes responsibility for coordination of radiological monitoring and assessment activities. (See the Recovery section of this annex for information on the FRMAC transfer.)

Some participating federal agencies have radiological planning and emergency responsibilities as part of their statutory authority. The monitoring and assessment activity coordinated by the FRMAC does not alter these responsibilities but complements them by providing for coordination of the federal radiological monitoring and assessment response activities.

- **DOE Aerial Measuring System (AMS)**—The DOE AMS characterizes ground-deposited radiation from aerial platforms. These platforms include fixed-wing and rotary-wing aircraft with radiological measuring equipment, computer analysis of aerial measurements, and equipment to locate lost radioactive sources, conduct aerial surveys, or map large areas of contamination.
- **DOE ARG**—The DOE ARG response element comprises scientists, technical specialists, crisis managers, and equipment ready to respond to the scene of a U.S. nuclear weapon accident to make the weapon safe for shipment.
- **DOE National Atmospheric Release Advisory Center (NARAC)**—The DOE NARAC provides a computer-based emergency preparedness and response predictive modeling capability. The NARAC is an off-site resource that supports the incident response remotely. The NARAC provides real-time computer predictions of the atmospheric transport of material from radioactive releases and of the downwind effects on health and safety. When measurement data become available, they are used to improve model predictions.
- **DOE Radiation Emergency Assistance Center/Training Site (REAC/TS)**—The DOE REAC/TS provides medical advice, specialized training, and on-site assistance for the treatment of all types of radiation exposure accidents. Additionally, through the Cytogenetic Biodosimetry Laboratory (CBL), REAC/TS provides for postexposure evaluation of radiation dose received.
- **DOE Radiological Assistance Program (RAP) Team**—DOE RAP teams are located at various DOE Operations Offices, Site Offices, and

National Laboratories. They can be dispatched to a radiological incident from Regional DOE Offices in response to a radiological incident. The RAP teams provide first-responder radiological assistance to protect the health and safety of the general public, responders, and the environment and to assist in the detection, identification and analysis, and response to events that involve radiological/nuclear material. Deployed RAP teams provide traditional field monitoring and assessment support as well as a search capability.

- **Nuclear Incident Response Team (NIRT)**—The NIRT consists of (1) the DOE resources described above and (2) EPA entities that perform such support functions (including radiological emergency response functions) and related functions. Under the Homeland Security Act of 2002, DHS has the authority to activate NIRT assets. When activated, the NIRT operates under DHS direction, authority, and control. When not operating as part of the NIRT, these assets remain under the control of the parent agency.

- **The Interagency Modeling and Atmospheric Assessment Center (IMAAC)**—The IMAAC is an interagency center responsible for production, coordination, and dissemination of the federal consequence predictions for an airborne hazardous material release. Through a partnership of the Departments of Homeland Security, Energy, Defense, and Commerce [through the National Oceanic and Atmospheric Administration (NOAA)], EPA, NASA, and NRC, the IMAAC provides the single federal atmospheric prediction of hazardous material concentration to all levels of the incident command. The IMAAC is an off-site resource that supports the incident response remotely. The NARAC is the interim IMAAC.

- **Advisory Team for Environment, Food, and Health**—The Advisory Team includes representatives from EPA, the U.S. Department of Agriculture (USDA), the Food and Drug Administration (FDA), the Centers for Disease Control (CDC) and Prevention, and other federal agencies. The advisory team develops coordinated advice and recommendations on environmental, food, health, and animal health matters for the Incident Command/Unified Command (IC/UC), DHS, the Joint Federal Office (JFO) Unified Coordination Group, the coordinating agency, and/or state, tribal, and local governments, as appropriate. The advisory team uses information provided by the IMAAC, FRMAC, and other relevant sources. The advisory team provides federal advice in matters related to the following:
  - Environmental assessments (field monitoring) required for developing recommendations with advice from state, tribal, and local governments and/or the FRMAC

- PAGs and their application to the emergency
- Protective action recommendations (PARs) using data and assessment from the FRMAC
- Protective actions to prevent or minimize contamination of milk, food, and water, and to prevent or minimize exposure through ingestion
- Recommendations for minimizing losses of agricul tural resources from radiation effects
- Availability of food, animal feed, and water supply inspection programs to ensure wholesomeness
- Relocation, reentry, and other radiation protection measures prior to recovery
- Recommendations for recovery, return, and cleanup issues
- Health and safety advice or information for the public and for workers
- Estimated effects of radioactive releases on human health and the environment
- Other matters, as requested by the IC or coordinating agency

- **EPA Radiological Emergency Response Team (RERT)**—The EPA RERT provides resources, including personnel, specialized equipment, technical expertise, and laboratory services to aid coordinating and cooperating agencies and state, tribal, and local response organizations in protecting the public and the environment from unnecessary exposure to ionizing radiation from radiological incidents. The RERT is a designated Special Team under the NCP. It may become part of the FRMAC if one is established. The RERT provides the following:
  - Monitoring, sampling, laboratory analyses, and data assessments using field emergency response assets
  - Technical advice and assistance for containment, cleanup, restoration, and recovery following a radiological incident
  - Assistance in the development and long-term recovery plans
  - Coordination with fixed laboratory assets for in-depth analysis and evaluation of large numbers of site-specific emergency response samples

- **EPA RadNet**—The EPA RadNet comprises a system of fixed and deployable radiation monitoring stations. The RadNet fixed monitoring stations provide a nationwide environmental monitoring network for the assessment of nationwide impacts from a radiological incident. The deployable component can provide site-specific emergency monitoring for more assessment of localized impacts during radiological emergencies. Although other assets can be used in nuclear/radiological incidents, their primary function is addressed elsewhere in the NRF or the annexes; see the Nuclear/Radiological Incident Annex.

E.6 CONCEPT OF OPERATIONS

This concept of operations is applicable to potential and actual radiological/ nuclear incidents requiring federal coordination as delineated in this annex.

E.6.1 General

The owner/operator of a nuclear/radiological facility or materials (e.g., DOE, DOD, or NRC licensee) primarily is responsible for mitigating the consequences of an incident; providing notification and appropriate protective action recommendations to state, local, and/or tribal government officials; and minimizing the radiological hazard to the public. For incidents that involve fixed facilities, the owner/operator has primary responsibility for actions within the facility boundary and may also have responsibilities for response and recovery activities outside the facility boundary under applicable legal obligations (e.g., contractual, licensee, CERCLA). For areas surrounding a nuclear/radiological incident location, the state, tribal, and local governments have primary responsibility for protecting life, property, and the environment. This does not, however, relieve nuclear/radiological facility or material owners/operators from applicable legal obligations.

State, tribal, and local governments as well as the owners/operators of nuclear/radiological facilities or activities should request assistance through established regulatory communication and response protocols. However, they may request assistance directly from DHS, other federal agencies, and/ or state governments with which they have preexisting arrangements or relationships, providing that the agency with regulatory authority is also notified.

State, tribal, and local governments are encouraged to integrate their radiological monitoring and assessment activities with the FRMAC.

E.6.2 Notification

The owner/operator of a nuclear/radiological facility or owner/transporter of nuclear/radiological material is generally the first to become aware of an incident and notifies state, tribal, and local authorities and the coordinating agency.

Federal, State, tribal, and local governments that become aware of a radiological incident should notify the coordinating agency and the DHS National Operations Center (NOC) at 202-282-8101 and comply with other appropriate statutory requirements for notification. For example, releases of reportable quantities of any listed hazardous materials as described within 40 CFR Part

302 must be reported to the National Response Center at 800-424-8802. Furthermore, state, tribal, and local law enforcement agencies should continue to contact the local FBI/Joint Terrorism Task Force regarding ongoing terrorist activities, events, instances, or investigations. The coordinating agency provides notification of a radiological incident to the NOC and other federal agencies, as appropriate. If a state requests radiological assistance directly from a federal agency for a nuclear/radiological incident that falls under the jurisdiction of another coordinating agency, that federal agency shall notify the coordinating agency of the request.

E.6.3   Activation

Once notified, the coordinating agency initiates response in accordance with its authorities. The DHS reviews the situation and determines whether to assume federal leadership for the overall response in accordance with the NRF. Coordinating agencies and cooperating agencies provide representatives to the NRF elements (e.g., JFO, NOC, etc.) when appropriate. For Stafford Act incidents, DHS/FEMA may issue mission assignments to federal agencies to support such activities.

If the DHS does not assume federal leadership for the response, a coordinating agency may request that the DHS activate NRF elements to support the response. The coordinating agency may request assistance from other federal agencies.

The coordinating agency also will be represented in appropriate positions within the Command Staff in the IC/UC structure (as defined by NIMS), and coordinates federal radiological response activities at appropriate field facilities.[6] Coordinating agencies and cooperating agencies provide personnel to other sections of the IC/UC as needed.

For any nuclear/radiological incident, the coordinating and cooperating agencies may establish a field facility; assist state, tribal, and local response organizations; monitor and support owner/operator activities (when there is an owner or operator); provide technical support to the owner/operator, if requested; and serve as a federal source of information about incident conditions.

Table E.3 below summarizes the activation process for some of the key federal radiological/nuclear assets.

---

[6]Appropriate field facilities may include an Incident/Area Command Post, Emergency Operations Center, Emergency Operations Facility, Emergency Control Center, and so on.

TABLE E.3   Activation of Key Assets for Nuclear/Radiological Incidents

Asset	Activation Process
IMAAC	The DHS, coordinating agencies, and the authorized IMAAC requestors (as designated in the IMAAC Standard Operating Procedures) may request IMAAC activation directly from the IMAAC or from the NOC Watch at 202-282-8101.
	The NOC Watch ensures that federal agencies are notified when the IMAAC has been activated for the purpose of generating the single and interagency coordinated federal prediction of atmospheric dispersions and their consequences.
Advisory Team	DHS, coordinating agencies, and state, tribal, and local governments may request support from the Advisory Team by contacting the CDC Director's Emergency Operations Center (EOC) at 770-488-7100.
	The DOE will request activation of the Advisory Team whenever the FRMAC is activated.
FRMAC and DOE Assets (AMS, ARG, RAP, REAC/TS, NARAC, and CMHT)	Coordinating agencies and state, tribal, and local governments may request a FRMAC or other support from the DOE or DHS. The FRMAC and all other DOE National Nuclear Security Administration (NNSA) assets may be requested through the DOE 24-hour Watch Office at 202-586-8100.
	Requests for RAP teams may also be directed to the appropriate Regional DOE Office.
	The DOE may respond to a request for assistance by initially dispatching an RAP team. If the situation requires more assistance than a RAP team can provide, then the DOE alerts or activates additional resources.
NIRT	The NIRT is activated when the DHS, in consultation with the EPA and DOE, determines that the severity of an incident warrants the NIRT assets. The NOC will notify the EPA and DOE when the NIRT is activated.
RERT	The DHS and coordinating agencies may request support from the EPA RERT by contacting the National Response Center at 800-424-8802.

E.6.4   ICS Implementation

The initial response to domestic incidents is typically handled at the local level. Local responders are responsible for implementing an Incident Command System (ICS) to manage the incident response. Federal agencies will integrate into the IC in support of the local jurisdictions. Most incidents under this annex will be multiagency/multijurisdictional responses, and the ICS Command function will be managed by a UC.

The coordinating agency is expected to participate in the IC/UC at the highest level (e.g., at the Area Command level if established). Other agencies may also participate in the IC/UC when consistent with ICS principles.

The key federal radiological assets will integrate into the IC/UC as appropriate. Specifically, the RAP team incorporates into the Operations Section of the IC/UC. Because the primary function of the FRMAC is to provide information for planning incident response operations, planning for FRMAC activities is expected to incorporate into IC/UC in the Planning Section, which is consistent with ICS principles. FRMAC personnel will work within the ICS to develop the Monitoring and Sampling Plan and to ensure that it is reflected in and consistent with the Incident Action Plan (IAP). The AMS normally reports to the FRMAC and operates in accordance with the IAP. The FRMAC structure will remain flexible and will be tailored to specific incident requirements.

During the initial phases of the incident, when the DOE is responsible for the FRMAC, it will be established organizationally as a discrete unit within the IC/UC structure to coordinate all radiological monitoring and assessment activities in support of state, tribal, and local authorities, the coordinating agency, and the DHS.

The advisory team is expected to integrate into the Planning Section to provide technical expertise to the IC/UC and coordinating agency. The advisory team may also provide liaisons to and/or coordinate with the JFO and state, tribal, and local government EOCs, as needed.

E.7   RESPONSE ACTIVITIES

Table E.4 presents the specific capabilities and responsibilities carried out by coordinating agencies and cooperating agencies to support state, tribal, and local activities during the response.

TABLE E.4 Nuclear/Radiological Incident Response Activities

Response Activity	Federal Agency Capabilities/Responsibilities
Incident Security	• The DOD, DOE, or NASA may establish NDAs or NSAs for special nuclear materials under their control, to safeguard classified information and/or restricted data, or equipment and material, and place nonfederal lands under federal control for the duration of the incident the DOD, DOE, or NASA, as appropriate, coordinates security in and around these locations, as necessary. • For incidents at other federal or private facilities, the owner/operator provides security within the facility boundaries. If a release of radioactive material occurs beyond the facility boundaries, then state, tribal, or local governments provide security for the release area. • State, tribal, and local governments provide security for radiological incidents that occur on public lands (e.g., a transportation incident) other than within NDAs or NSAs. • ESF #13—Public Safety and Security may be activated to provide additional security resources and capabilities (e.g., for an RDD/IND).
Unknown Material Identification	The DHS Domestic Nuclear Detection Office (DNDO) Joint Analysis Center (JAC) may respond to a state, tribal, local, or coordinating agency request for assistance in identifying an unknown nuclear/radiological material. The DNDO coordinates the technical adjudication of a radiation detection alarm and recommends technical federal asset responses as required.
Atmospheric Plume Modeling	• When the DHS coordinates the overall federal response, the IMAAC generates the single and interagency coordinated federal prediction of atmospheric dispersions and their consequences. The IMAAC predictions are used for risk management decisions, public information, and operational response. The IMAAC may also generate predictions for other incidents that require federal coordination. • Plume models are initially generated using default assumptions and then are refined over time as actual data from on-scene responders become available.

(Continued)

TABLE E.4 *Continued*

Response Activity	Federal Agency Capabilities/Responsibilities
	• The coordinating agency is responsible for ensuring the outputs from the IMAAC are shared with all appropriate response organizations.
Environmental Monitoring and Sampling for Characterization and Reentry	• Federal responders may provide radiological monitoring and assessment data directly to state, tribal, and local governments as requested in support of protective action decision making.
	• If the FRMAC is not stood up, then the coordinating agency assumes responsibility for coordinating the federal monitoring and assessment activities with state, tribal, and local governments. Support may be provided to the coordinating agency by ESF #10 when appropriate.
	• When an FRMAC is established, the FRMAC assumes responsibility for coordinating federal monitoring and assessment activities. The DOE will provide a mechanism for transmitting data to and from the FRMAC within NIMS/ICS protocols. Until the FRMAC is operational, federal first responders continue to provide data directly to state, tribal, and local governments, and coordinate radiological monitoring and assessment data with the DOE Consequence Management Home Team (CMHT) or the Consequence Management Response Team (CMRT).
	• When requested, the DOE and other federal agencies may provide radiation safety support for reentry to critical infrastructure and for other critical activities.
	• The coordinating agency is responsible for ensuring that all outputs from the FRMAC are shared with all appropriate response organizations.
	• The DOE initially has the FRMAC lead, but the FRMAC lead will transition to EPA for recovery/remediation.
	• For incidents that involve terrorism, any participating federal agency may raise issues regarding the sharing of sensitive data for responder and public safety that cannot be resolved at the Incident Command level to the Unified Coordination Group for resolution.

(Continued)

TABLE E.4 *Continued*

Response Activity	Federal Agency Capabilities/Responsibilities
Emergency Worker Monitoring	• Each response agency has the responsibility to monitor the safety of its own workers. • The Occupational Safety and Health Administration provides support and regulatory oversight, as necessary, through the Worker Safety and Health Support Annex.
Protective Action Recommendations	• Federal PARs may include advice and assistance on measures to avoid or reduce exposure of the public to radiation from a release of radioactive material. This includes advice on emergency actions such as sheltering, evacuation, prophylactic use of potassium iodide, and administration of other pharmaceutical countermeasures. It also includes advice on long-term measures, such as food restrictions, temporary relocation, or permanent resettlement, to avoid or minimize exposure to residual radiation or exposure through the ingestion pathway. • Data in support of health and safety will be shared among response agencies prior to the development of formal PARs. Incident-specific federal PARs are developed by the advisory team and are largely based on the EPA's PAGs for radiological incidents. • Federal PARs are coordinated through the IC/UC (which includes the coordinating agency) and multiagency coordination groups. The coordinating agency is responsible for ensuring that all outputs from the advisory team are shared with appropriate response organizations. • State, tribal, and local governments are responsible for implementing protective actions as they deem appropriate.
Population Monitoring	• The Department of Health and Human Services (HHS), through ESF #8—Public Health and Medical Services and in consultation with the coordinating agency, coordinates federal support for external monitoring of people. • HHS assists local and state health departments in establishing a registry of potentially exposed individuals, performing dose reconstruction, and conducting long-term monitoring of this population for potential long-term health effects.

(Continued)

TABLE E.4 *Continued*

Response Activity	Federal Agency Capabilities/Responsibilities
Laboratory Analysis	Federal agencies provide laboratory capabilities for certain types of analyses. Examples of capabilities include the FDA (HHS) for food and agriculture analysis; the CDC (HHS) for bioassays; and the EPA and DOE for environmental samples.
Environmental Monitoring and Sampling for Cleanup Verification	• The responsibility for this activity is defined by applicable laws and regulations, and is typically the responsibility of nuclear/radiological facility and material owners and operators. • The EPA may provide support under ESF #10 when appropriate.
Release of Public Information	For incidents in which the DHS leads the overall federal response (under HSPD-5), DHS/ESF #15—External Affairs coordinates the release of federal public information regarding the incident. Otherwise, the coordinating agency is responsible for the release of federal public information.
Population Decontamination	• The decontamination of possibly affected victims is accomplished locally and is the responsibility of state, tribal, and local governments. • Federal resources are provided at the request of, and in support of, the affected state(s). HHS, through ESF #8 and in consultation with the coordinating agency, coordinates federal support for population decontamination. • The HHS assists and supports state, tribal, and local governments in performing monitoring for internal contamination and administering available pharmaceuticals for internal decontamination, as deemed necessary by state health officials.
Emergency Worker Decontamination	• The FRMAC provides support for the decontamination of federal, state, and local emergency responders integrating into the FRMAC. • Agencies are responsible for decontamination of their own workers not integrated in the FRMAC.
Response Equipment Decontamination	• The FRMAC provides support for the decontamination of federal, state, and local equipment integrating into the FRMAC.

(Continued)

TABLE E.4   *Continued*

Response Activity	Federal Agency Capabilities/Responsibilities
	• Agencies are responsible for decontamination of their own equipment that is not integrated in the FRMAC.
Fatality Management	Fatality management is primarily a state responsibility. The HHS coordinates the federal support to the states.
Contaminated Animal Management	• The USDA provides support for the assessment, control, and decontamination of contaminated animals, including companion animals, livestock, poultry, and wildlife. • The USDA provides support for the stabilization and disposition of contaminated animal carcasses, with additional support from ESF #3—Public Works and Engineering and ESF #10.
Contaminated Agricultural Product Management	USDA provides support under ESF #11— Agriculture and Natural Resources, with additional support from ESF #3 and ESF #10 for the assessment, stabilization, and disposal of contaminated animal products and plant materials including food, feed, fiber, and crops.
Radioactive Waste Storage and Disposal	• The responsibility for this activity is defined by applicable laws and regulations, and it is typically the responsibility of nuclear/radiological facility and material owners and operators. • The EPA may provide support under ESF #10 when appropriate. • The DOD/USACE and other federal agencies may provide additional support as needed for RDD/IND incidents.
Contaminated Debris Removal	• The responsibility for this activity is defined by applicable laws and regulations, and it is typically the responsibility of nuclear/radiological facility and material owners and operators. • Support is provided as a joint effort between ESF #3 (DOD/USACE) and ESF #10 (EPA).
Environmental Remediation	• Responsibility for this activity is defined by applicable laws and regulations, and is typically the responsibility of nuclear/radiological facility and material owners and operators. • EPA may provide support under ESF #10 when appropriate. • DOD/USACE and other federal agencies may provide additional support as needed for RDD/IND incidents.

E.8 RECOVERY

When the DHS is coordinating the federal response, it coordinates, in concert with cognizant state, tribal, and local governments, overall federal recovery pursuant to the NRF. The coordinating agency maintains responsibility for managing the federal technical radiological cleanup activities in accordance with its statutory authorities, responsibilities, and NRF mechanisms.

For all other radiological incidents, the coordinating agency coordinates environmental remediation/cleanup in concert with cognizant state, tribal, and local governments, as well as owners/operators, as applicable. While retaining the technical lead for these activities, the coordinating agency may request support from a cooperating agency that has cleanup/recovery experience and capabilities (e.g., EPA and USACE). State, tribal, and local governments primarily are responsible for planning the recovery of the affected area. (The term "recovery," as used here, encompasses any action dedicated to the continued protection of the public and resumption of normal activities in the affected area.) Recovery planning generally does not take place until the initiating conditions of the incident have stabilized and immediate actions to protect public health, safety, and property are accomplished. On request, the federal government assists state, tribal, and local governments with developing and executing recovery plans. Private owners/operators have primary responsibility for recovery planning activities and eventual cleanup within their facility boundaries and may have responsibilities for recovery activities outside their facility under applicable legal obligations (e.g., contractual, licensee, and CERCLA).

The DOE FRMAC Director works closely with the FRMAC's Senior EPA representative to facilitate a smooth transition of the federal radiological monitoring and assessment coordination responsibility to the EPA at a mutually agreeable time, and after consultation with the DHS; the Unified Coordination Group; and state, tribal, and local governments. The following conditions are intended to be met prior to transfer:

- The immediate emergency condition is stabilized.
- Off-site releases of radioactive material have ceased, and there is little or no potential for further unintentional off-site releases.
- The off-site radiological conditions are evaluated, and the immediate consequences are assessed.
- An initial long-range monitoring plan has been developed in conjunction with the affected state, tribal, and local governments and appropriate federal agencies.

TABLE E.5   Additional federal Agency Capabilities for a
Nuclear/Radiological Incident

Agency	Capabilities
Department of Agriculture	(See the ESF #11 Annex and the Food and Agriculture Incident Annex for additional USDA responsibilities).
	• Assists in the planning and collection of agricultural samples within the Ingestion Exposure Pathway Emergency Planning Zone.
	• Assesses damage to crops, soil, livestock, poultry, and processing facilities and incorporates the findings in a damage assessment report.
	• Assists in the evaluation and assessment of data to determine the impact of the incident on agriculture.
	• Provides support and advice on the screening and decontamination of pets and farm animals that may have been exposed to radiation or contaminated with radioactive materials.
	• Assists in the planning and operational aspects of animal carcasses disposal.
	• Inspects and assists in the collection of samples of crops, meat and meat products, poultry and poultry products, and egg products to ensure that they are safe for human consumption.
	• Assists, in conjunction with the HHS, in monitoring the production, processing, storage, and distribution of food through the wholesale level to eliminate contaminated product and to ensure that the levels of contamination in the product are safe and below the derived intervention levels (DILs).
Department of Commerce	• Provides near or on-scene weather observations on request.
	• Prepares forecasts tailored to support emergency incident management activities.
	• Participates in the IMAAC by providing atmospheric transport and dispersion (plume) modeling assessment and forecasts, surface weather observations, and weather forecasts to the IMAAC, when activated.
	• When the IMAAC is not activated, it provides atmospheric transport and dispersion (plume) modeling assessment and forecasts to the coordinating agency, in accordance with established procedures.

(Continued)

TABLE E.5 *Continued*

Agency	Capabilities
	• Maintains and develops the HYSPLIT transport and dispersion model. • Archives, as a special collection, the meteorological data from national observing and numerical weather analysis and prediction systems applicable to the monitoring and assessment of the response. • Provides assistance and reference material for calibrating radiological instruments. • Provides support in the testing and evaluation of radiation shielding materials. • In the event of materials potentially crossing international boundaries, it provides atmospheric transport and dispersion products to international hydrometeorological services and associated agencies through the mechanisms afforded by the World Meteorological Organization. • Provides radioanalytical measurement support and instrumentation. • Provides assistance for collection and monitoring for marine and estuary contamination assessment. • Advises and provides assistance on building operations (e.g., HVAC) for contamination control and decontamination processes. • Provides laboratory support for the analysis of materials and environmental samples.
Department of Defense	• Provides Defense Support of Civil Authorities (DSCA) in response to requests for assistance during domestic incidents. With the exception of support provided under the Immediate Response Authority, the obligation of DOD resources to support requests for assistance is subject to the approval of the Secretary of Defense. Under certain critical circumstances, the President or Secretary of Defense may direct DSCA activities without a specific request. Details regarding DSCA and immediate response are provided in the NRF Core Document. • Provides DSCA in response to requests for assistance during domestic incidents. With the exception of support provided under Immediate Response Authority, the obligation of DOD resources to support requests for

TABLE E.5   *Continued*

Agency	Capabilities
	assistance is subject to the approval of the Secretary of Defense. Under certain critical circumstances, the President or Secretary of Defense may direct DSCA activities without a specific request. Details regarding DSCA and immediate response are provided in the NRF Core Document. • May provide DOD and DOD-funded assets for the response to radiological incidents, to include the following. • Weapons of Mass Destruction Civil Support Teams (WMD CSTs)—National Guard teams that assess a suspected WMD attack, advise civilian responders on appropriate actions through on-site testing and expert reachback, and facilitate the arrival of additional state and federal military forces. Each team consists of 22 personnel and is equipped with personal protective equipment for operating in unknown hazardous environments, NBC (nuclear, biological, and chemical) detectors, sampling/analytical systems, a decontamination system, and communications equipment used to reach back to experts via satellite. These state assets can be federalized. There is nominally one CST per state, as well as one each in Guam, Puerto Rico, the Virgin Islands, and the District of Columbia. • CBRN (chemical, biological, radiological, and nuclear) Enhanced Response Force Packages (CERFPs)—National Guard elements that provide an immediate response capability to a Governor. The CERFPs are capable of searching an incident site (including damaged buildings), rescuing any casualties, decontaminating them, and performing medical triage and initial treatment to stabilize them for transport to a medical facility. This includes extracting anyone trapped in the rubble. The CERFP is composed of four elements staffed by personnel from already established National Guard units. The elements are search and extraction, decontamination, medical, and security. The CERFP command and control team directs the overall activities of the CERFP and coordinates with the Joint Task Force—State

TABLE E.5 *Continued*

Agency	Capabilities
	and the Incident Commander. There is at least one CERFP in each FEMA region.
	• CBRNE (chemical, biological, radiological, nuclear, and high-yield explosive) Consequence Management Response Forces (CCMRF)—Multi-service (active and reserve component military) follow-on assets designed to augment the CSTs and CERFPs, if necessary. Specific CCMRF capabilities include, but are not limited to, robust command and control, technical search and rescue, explosive ordnance disposal, aviation evacuation, specialized medical response teams, and enhanced chemical, biological, and nuclear detection/decontamination.
	• DOD advisory teams—Various teams that may deploy, either independently or as part of the CCMRFs, that provide guidance and advice to the Incident Commander on potential health hazards, radiation injury treatment, survey data evaluations, population monitoring, etc. These include the Consequence Management Advisory Team (CMAT), U.S. Air Force Radiation Assessment Team (AFRAT), the U.S. Army's Radiological Advisory Medical Team (RAMT), and the Armed Forces Radiobiology Research Institute's Medical Radiobiological Advisory Team (MRAT).
	• Provides immediate assistance under Immediate Response Authority for any civil emergency that may require immediate action to save lives, prevent human suffering, or mitigate great property damage. When such conditions exist and time does not permit prior approval from higher headquarters, local military commanders and responsible officials from DOD components and agencies are authorized by DOD directive, subject to any supplemental direction that may be provided by their DOD component, to take necessary action to respond to requests of civil authorities. All such necessary action is referred to as "Immediate Response."
Department of Defense/U.S. Army Corps of Engineers	(See the ESF #3—Public Works and Engineering Annex for additional information.)

(Continued)

TABLE E.5 *Continued*

Agency	Capabilities

	• For RDD/IND incidents, provides response and clean-up support as a cooperating agency.
	• Integrates and coordinates with other agencies, as requested, to perform any or all of the following:
	  • Radiological survey functions.
	  • Gross decontamination.
	  • Site characterization.
	  • Contaminated water and debris management.
	  • Site remediation.

Department of Energy	• Develops and maintains FRMAC policies and procedures, determines FRMAC composition, and maintains FRMAC operational readiness. • Coordinates federal radiological environmental monitoring and assessment activities as lead technical organization in the FRMAC (emergency phase), regardless of who is designated the coordinating agency. • Maintains technical liaison with state and local agencies with monitoring and assessment responsibilities. • Maintains a common set of all radiological monitoring data in an accountable, secure, and retrievable form and ensures the technical integrity of FRMAC data. • Provides monitoring data and interpretations, including exposure rate contours, dose projections, and any other requested radiological assessments, to the coordinating agency and to the states. • Provides, in cooperation with other federal agencies, the personnel and equipment to perform radiological monitoring and assessment activities, and provides on-scene analytical capability supporting assessments. • Requests supplemental assistance and technical support from other federal agencies as needed. • Arranges consultation and support services through appropriate federal agencies to all other entities (e.g., private contractors) with radiological monitoring functions and capabilities and technical and medical expertise for handling radiological contamination and population monitoring.

(Continued)

TABLE E.5   *Continued*

Agency	Capabilities
	• Works closely with the Senior EPA representative to facilitate a smooth transition of the federal radiological monitoring and assessment coordination responsibility to EPA at a mutually agreeable time and after consultation with the states and coordinating agency. • Provides, in cooperation with other federal and state agencies, personnel and equipment, including portal monitors, to support initial external screening and provides advice and assistance to state and local personnel conducting screening/decontamination of persons leaving a contaminated zone. • Provides plume trajectories and deposition projections from NARAC for emergency response. • Provides source term estimates to the IMAAC and/or coordinating agency when limited or no information is available, based on DOE's unique experience in developing source terms for INDs and RDDs. • Upgrades, maintains, coordinates, and publishes documentation needed for the administration, implementation, operation, and standardization of the FRMAC. • Maintains and improves the ability to provide wide-area radiation monitoring now resident in the AMS. • Maintains and improves the ability to provide medical assistance, advisory teams, and training related to nuclear/radiological accidents and incidents now resident in the REAC/TS. • Maintains and improves the ability to provide predictive modeling of airborne hazards and to correct modeled results through integration of actual radiation measurements obtained from both airborne and ground sources, resident in the FRMAC. The NARAC maintains and improves their ability to model the direct results (blast, thermal, radiation, and EMP) of a nuclear detonation. • Maintains and improves the first-response ability to assess an emergency situation and to advise decisionmakers on what further steps can be taken to evaluate and minimize the

(Continued)

TABLE E.5   *Continued*

Agency	Capabilities
	hazards of a radiological emergency resident in the RAP.
	• Maintains and improves the ability to respond to an emergency involving U.S. nuclear weapons resident in the ARG.
	• Maintains and improves the ability of CMHTs and CMRTs to provide initial planning, coordination, and data collection and assessment prior to or in lieu of establishment of a FRMAC.
	• Maintains and improves the ability of the DOE Nuclear/Radiological Advisory Team to provide advice and limited technical assistance, including search, diagnostics, and effects prediction, as part of a Domestic Emergency Support Team.
	• Maintains and improves the ability of Radiological Triage to determine, through remote analysis of nuclear spectra collected on-scene, if a radioactive object contains special nuclear materials.
	• Assigns a Senior Energy Official (SEO) for any response involving the deployment of the DOE/NNSA emergency response assets. The SEO will integrate into an appropriate position in the IC/UC and is responsible for the coordination and employment of these assets at the scene of a radiological event. The deployed assets will work in support of and under the direction of the SEO.
Department of Health and Human Services	(See the ESF #8 Annex for additional information.)
	• Conducts epidemiological surveillance and provides guidance on methods to detect symptoms consistent with exposure to radioactive materials.
	• Collects samples of agricultural products to monitor and assess the extent of contamination as a basis for recommending or implementing protective actions (through the FRMAC).
	• Provides advice on proper medical treatment of the general population and response workers exposed to or contaminated by radioactive materials.

(Continued)

TABLE E.5 *Continued*

Agency	Capabilities
	• Provides available medical countermeasures through deployment of the Strategic National Stockpile. • Provides assessment and treatment teams for those exposed to or contaminated by radiation. • Provides advice and guidance in assessing the impact of the effects of radiological incidents on the health of persons in the affected area. • Manages long-term public monitoring and supports follow-on personal data collection, collecting and processing of blood samples and bodily fluids/matter samples, and advice concerning medical assessment and triage of victims. Tracks patient treatment and long-term health effects.
Department of Homeland Security/Customs and Border Protection	• For incidents at the border, maintains radiation detection equipment and nonintrusive inspection technology at ports of entry and Border Patrol checkpoints to detect the presence of radiological substances transported by persons, cargo, mail, or conveyance arriving from foreign countries. • Through its National Targeting Center, provides extensive analytical and targeting capabilities to identify and interdict suspect nuclear/radiological materials. • Through the CBP Weapons of Mass Destruction Teleforensic Center, provides 24/7 support to DHS/CBP and other federal law enforcement personnel in the identification of interdicted suspect hazardous material as well as providing a link for coordination with and triage to other federal agencies as appropriate for the type of incident. • Through the CBP Laboratories and Scientific Services (LSS), staffs WMD Response Teams in strategic locations nationwide to screen and identify potential radiological threat materials as well as reduce the hazards that may exist by establishing temporary containment parameters.
Department of Homeland Security/Domestic Nuclear Detection Office (DNDO)	• Supports the deployment of an enhanced global nuclear detection system to detect and report on attempts to import, possess, store,

(Continued)

TABLE E.5 *Continued*

Agency	Capabilities
	transport, develop, or use an unauthorized nuclear explosive device, fissile material, or radiological material in the United States.
	• Through the DNDO Joint Analysis Center, provides a coordinated technical adjudication of a nuclear/radiation detection alarm, and recommends technical federal asset responses as required.
Department of Homeland Security/Federal Emergency Management Agency	Serves as the annex coordinator for this annex.
Department of Homeland Security/U.S. Coast Guard	• Because of its unique maritime jurisdiction and capabilities, is prepared to provide appropriate security, command and control, transportation, and support to other agencies that need to operate in the maritime domain.
	• Maintains the National Response Center, which is staffed by Coast Guard personnel who maintain a 24-hour-a-day, 365-day-a-year telephone watch.
Department of the Interior (DOI)	• Provides resources, including personnel, equipment, and laboratory support, to advise and assist in evaluating processes affecting radioisotopes in soils.
	• Provides resources, including personnel and equipment, to advise and assist in the development of geographic information systems databases to be used in the analysis and assessment of contaminated areas.
	• Provides liaison between federally recognized tribal governments and federal, State, and local agencies for coordination of response activities. Additionally, DOI advises and assists DHS on economic, social, and political matters in the U.S. insular areas should a radiological incident occur in these areas.
Department of Justice/Federal Bureau of Investigation	• Has lead responsibility for criminal investigations of terrorist acts or terrorist threats by individuals or groups inside the United States, or directed at U.S. citizens or institutions abroad, where such acts are within the federal criminal jurisdiction of the United States.
	• Manages, leads, and coordinates all law enforcement and investigative activities with

(Continued)

TABLE E.5 *Continued*

Agency	Capabilities
	regard to the response to terrorist acts or threats, including tactical operations, crime scene investigation, crisis negotiation, and intelligence gathering and dissemination.
	• Coordinates the activities of the law enforcement community to detect, prevent, preempt, and disrupt terrorist attacks against the United States.
	Additional details regarding the FBI response are outlined in the Terrorism Incident Law Enforcement and Investigation Annex.
Department of Labor/Occupational Safety and Health Administration	• Provides advice and technical assistance to DHS, the coordinating agency, and State, tribal, and local governments concerning the health and safety of response workers implementing the policies and concepts in this annex.
	• Provides assistance with developing site health and safety plans.
	• Provides monitoring for emergency response workers through the Worker Safety and Health Support Annex.
	• Provides technical assistance with emergency worker decontamination.
Department of State	• Serves as the U.S. Government lead in notification of the International Atomic Energy Agency (IAEA) in accordance with the Convention on Early Notification of a Nuclear Accident.
	• Serves as the U.S. Government lead in notification to foreign governments. Will immediately notify Canada and Mexico to negotiate cooperative and collaborative cross-border activities.
	• Serves as the U.S. Government lead in requesting or accepting assistance in accordance with the IAEA Convention on Assistance in Case of a Nuclear Accident or Radiological Emergency.
Department of Transportation	(See the ESF #1—Transportation Annex for further information.)
	Provides technical advice and assistance on the transportation of radiological materials and the impact of the incident on the transportation infrastructure.

(Continued)

TABLE E.5 *Continued*

Agency	Capabilities
Department of Veterans Affairs	Provides medical assistance using the Medical Emergency Radiological Response Team, which provides direct patient treatment; assists and trains local health care providers in managing, handling, and treatment of radiation-exposed and -contaminated casualties; assesses the impact on human health; and provides consultation and technical advice to local, state, and federal authorities.
Environmental Protection Agency	(See the ESF #10 Annex for additional information.) • Provides resources, including personnel, equipment, and laboratory support (including mobile laboratories) to assist DOE in monitoring radioactivity levels in the environment. • Assists in the development and implementation of a long-term monitoring plan and long-term recovery plan. • Provides nationwide environmental monitoring data from the RadNet for assessing the national impact of the incident. • Develops PAG manuals in coordination with the FRPCC. • Recommends acceptable emergency levels of radioactivity and radiation in the environment. • Prepares health and safety advice and information for the public. • Estimates effects of radioactive releases on human health and the environment. • Provides, in cooperation with other federal agencies, the law enforcement personnel and equipment to conduct law enforcement operations and investigations for nuclear/radiological incidents involving criminal activity that are not terrorism related.
National Aeronautics and Space Administration	• Partners with DOE when preparing for the launch of spacecraft involving significant quantities of DOE-owned nuclear material by providing additional specialized radiological monitoring equipment and radiological accident response personnel. However, NASA Centers maintain limited quantities of

(Continued)

TABLE E.5 *Continued*

Agency	Capabilities
	radiological monitoring equipment that could be used in response to radiological incidents. • In conjunction with EPA and NOAA, may task certain NASA orbiting assets to provide supplemental data to monitor incidents occurring in Earth's atmosphere.
Nuclear Regulatory Commission	• Provides technical assistance to include source term estimation, plume dispersion, and dose assessment calculations. • Provides assistance in federal radiological monitoring and assessment activities.

- The EPA has received adequate assurances from the other federal agencies that they are committing the required resources, personnel, and funds for the duration of the federal response.

Radiological monitoring and assessment activities are normally terminated when the coordinating agency, in consultation with other participating agencies and state, tribal, and local governments, determines the following:

- There is no longer a threat to public health and safety or the environment.
- State, tribal, and local resources are adequate for the situation.
- There is mutual agreement among the agencies involved to terminate monitoring and assessment.

E.9 FEDERAL CAPABILITIES AND ASSETS

In addition to leading specific portions of a response, coordinating agencies, along with other federal agencies, may bring specific expertise pertinent to nuclear/radiological incidents. Table E.5 below identifies the specific support that these agencies may provide.

APPENDIX F

POTENTIAL ISOTOPES LIKELY TO BE USED IN A RADIOLOGICAL DISPERSION DEVICE

Source: IAEA Categorization of radiation sources; March 2001;
IAEA-TECDOC-1191

Radioactive sources can be categorized by source type. Essentially categories are based on the use of the radioactive material and on the activity levels contained in them. The IAEA has ranked sources in general categories in the following manner:

Category 1   Industrial radiography
             Teletherapy
             Irradiators
Category 2   High dose rate (HDR) brachytherapy
             Fixed industrial gauges involving high activity sources
             Well logging
             Low dose rate (LDR) brachytherapy
Category 3   Fixed industrial gauges involving lower activity sources

Category 1 sources present significant hazards that require close scrutiny of the conditions of use, the construction and operation of the facility, the

Radiation Safety: Protection and Management for Homeland Security and Emergency Response. By L. A. Burchfield
Copyright © 2009 John Wiley & Sons, Inc.

training and competence of users, and the control mechanisms that the user will apply to assure safety and security. In general, a detailed safety assessment would be expected to support the authorization of the source or device, and also of the facility when the use is in a fixed location.

Category 1

Categorization of Radiation Sources: Information Concerning Practices and Radioactive Materials

Application	Isotope	Decay Mode Decay Energy [keV] Half-Life[a]	Activity Range	Dose Rate at 1 m [mSv/h]	Time at 1 m to Exceed 1 mSv
Teletherapy	Cobalt-60	γ (1173; 1333) β (max.: 318)	50–400 TBq	8E + 04	<1 second
	Cesium-137	T1/2 = 5.3 a γ (662) β (max.: 512) T1/2 = 30 a	500 TBq	3E + 04	<1 second
Blood irradiation	Cesium-137	T1/2 = 5.3 a γ (662) β (max.: 512) T1/2 = 30 a	2–100 TBq	6E + 03	<1 second
Industrial radiography	Iridium-192	γ (317) β (max.: 675) T1/2 = 74 days	0.1–4 TBq	4E + 02	9 second
	Cobalt-60	γ (1173; 1333) β (max.: 318) T1/2 = 5.3 a	0.1–5 TBq	1E + 03	3 second
	(Cesium-137) (rare)	γ (662) β (max.: 512) T1/2 = 30 a			
	(Thulium-170) (rare)	γ (84) β (max.: 968) T1/2 = 129 days			
Sterilization and food preservation (irradiators)	Cobalt-60	γ (1173; 1333) β (max.: 318) T1/2 = 5.3 a	0.1–400 PBq	1E + 08	<1 second
	Cesium-137	γ (662) β (max.: 512) T1/2 = 30 a	0.1–400 PBq	2E + 07	<1 second

Application	Isotope	Decay Mode Decay Energy [keV] Half-Life[a]	Activity Range	Dose Rate at 1 m [mSv/h]	Time at 1 m to Exceed 1 mSv
Other irradiators	Cobalt-60	γ (1173; 1333) β (max.: 318) T1/2 = 5.3 a	1–1000 TBq	3E + 05	<1 second
	(Cesium-137) (rare)	γ (662) β (max.: 512) T1/2 = 30 a			<1 second

[a]*Abbreviation*: a = annum (years).

Category 2 sources may present significant hazards that will require examination, and the regulatory authority needs to be aware of issues such as patient protection, which have not been considered in this categorization. Although the quantities of radioactive material may be lower for sources in category 2, other source attributes, such as portability and accessibility, will remain critical, including the potential loss of accountability and the presence of reasonable options for the disposition of disused or spent sources.

Category 2

Application	Isotope	Decay Mode Decay Energy [keV] Half-Life[a]	Activity Range	Dose Rate at 1 m [mSv/h]	Time at 1 m to Exceed 1 mSv
Remote after loading brachy-therapy (high dose rate)	Cobalt-60	γ (1173; 1333) β (max.: 318) T1/2 = 5.3 a	≈10 GBq	3E + 00	20 minutes
	Iridium-192	γ (317) β (max.: 675) T1/2 = 74 days	≈400 GBq	3E + 01	2 minutes
Manual and remote brachytherapy (low dose rate)	Cesium-137	γ (662) β (max.: 512) T1/2 = 30 a	0.05–4 GBq	2E − 01	5 hours
	Radium-226	γ (186) α (4784) T1/2 = 1600 a	30–300 MBq	2E − 04	20 days

Application	Isotope	Decay Mode Decay Energy [keV] Half-Life[a]	Activity Range	Dose Rate at 1 m [mSv/h]	Time at 1 m to Exceed 1 mSv
	Cobalt-60	γ (1173; 1333) β (max.: 318) T1/2 = 5.3 a	50–500 MBq	1E − 01	8 hours
	Strontium-90	β (max.: 546) T1/2 = 29 a	50–1500 MBq	0	N/A
	Palladium-103	X (20) T1/2 = 17 days	50–1500 MBq	0	N/A
Well logging	Cesium-137	γ (662) β (max.: 512) T1/2 = 30 a	1–100 GBq	6E + 00	10 minutes
	Americium-241/ Beryllium	γ (60) α (5486) neutrons T1/2 = 432.2 a	1–800 GBq	2E + 00	30 minutes
	(Californium-252)	α (6118) X (15) T1/2 = 2.6 a neutrons	50 GBq	6E + 1 (neutrons)	1 minute
Level gauge Thickness gauge Conveyor gauge	Cesium-137	γ (662) β (max.: 512) T1/2 = 30 a	20–500 GBq	3E + 01	2 minutes
	Cobalt-60	γ (1173; 1333) β (max.: 318) T1/2 = 5.3 a	0.1–10 GBq	3E + 00	20 minutes
	Americium-241	γ (60) α (5486) T1/2 = 432.2 a	1–100 GBq	3E − 01	3 hours
Moisture/ density detector	Americium-241/ Beryllium	γ (60) α (5486) neutrons T1/2 = 432.2 a	0.1–2 GBq	6E − 03	7 days
	Cesium-137	γ (662) β (max.: 512) T1/2 = 30 a	to 400 MBq	2E − 02	2 days
	(Californium-252)	α (6118) X (15) T1/2 = 2.6 a Neutrons	3 GBq	4E + 00	15 minutes

Application	Isotope	Decay Mode Decay Energy [keV] Half-Life^a	Activity Range	Dose Rate at 1 m [mSv/h]	Time at 1 m to Exceed 1 mSv
	(Radium-226/ Beryllium)	γ (60) α (5486) T1/2 = 432.2 a neutrons	~1500 MBq		

^{a}*Abbreviation*: a = annum (years).

Category 3 sources will require less effort on the part of the regulatory authority. In many cases, safety and security during operations is a function of the device construction, and a detailed review of a particular application for use will not be needed. However, the regulatory authority will need to remain mindful of end-of-life issues where there may be the potential for a loss of regulatory control if accountability is not maintained.

Category 3

Application	Isotope	Decay Mode Decay Energy [keV] Half-Life^a	Activity Range	Dose Rate at 1 m [mSv/h]	Time at 1 m to Exceed 1 mSv
Level gauge Density gauge	Cesium-137	γ (662) β (max.: 512) T1/2 = 30 a	0.1 − 10 GBq	5E − 01	2 hours
	Cobalt-60	γ (1173; 1333) β (max.: 318) T1/2 = 5.3 a	0.1 − 10 GBq	3E + 00	20 minutes
Thickness gauge	Krypton-85	β (max.: 687) T1/2 = 10.8 a	0.1 − 50 GBq	1E − 02	4 days
	Americium- 241	γ (60) α (5486) T1/2 = 432.2 a	4 GBq	1E − 02	4 days
	Strontium-90	β (max.: 546) T1/2 = 29 a	0.1−4 GBq	0	
	Thallium-204	γ (69) β (max.: 763) T1/2 = 3.8 a	10 GBq	1E − 03	(weeks)

^{a}*Abbreviation*: a = annum (years).

BIBLIOGRAPHY

American Nuclear Society. "Nuclear Science & Technology: Crucial to Sustainable Development." http://www.ans.org. 1999. Accessed.

Armed Forces Radiobiology Research Institute. "Training for the Unthinkable." http://www.afrri.usuhs.mil. 2004. Accessed.

Barretto, Paulo M.C. "Strengthening Capabilities: Safe Use of Radiation Applications Beyond 2000." http://www.iaea.org. 1999. Accessed.

"The Basics of Radiation and Radiation Health Effects." http://www.doh.wa.gov. 2005. Accessed.

"Beneficial Uses of Radiation." http://www.nei.org. 2007. Accessed.

Berger, M.E.; Leonard, R.B.; Ricks, R.C.; Wiley, A.L.; Lowry, P.C.; Flynn, D.F. "Hospital Triage in the First 24 Hours after a Nuclear or Radiological Disaster." http://orise.orau.gov. Accessed.

Broderick, Mick. "From Atoms to Apocalypse: Film and the Nuclear Issue." *Nuclear Movies*. http://www.mcc.murdoch.edu.au. 1991. Accessed.

Cerveny, Jan T. "Treatment of Internal Radionuclide Contamination." http://www.afrri.usuhs.mil. 1988. Accessed.

Cerveny, Jan T.; MacVittie, Thomas J.; Young, Robert W. "Acute Radiation Syndrome in Humans." http://www.afrri.usuhs. 1989. Accessed.

Chernus, Ira. "Eisenhower: Faith and Fear in the Fifties." http://spot.colorado.edu. Accessed.

Radiation Safety: Protection and Management for Homeland Security and Emergency Response. By L. A. Burchfield
Copyright © 2009 John Wiley & Sons, Inc.

Department of Homeland Security. "Chemical, Biological, Radiological, and Nuclear Countermeasures." http://www.whitehouse.gov. Accessed.

Dicus, Greta Joy. "U.S. Perspectives on Safety & Security of Radioactive Sources." http://iaea.org. 1999. Accessed.

Donigan, Emily. "Decontamination in a Radiological Event." http://exercises. washingtonguard.org. 2007. Accessed.

Dons, Robert F.; Cerveny, Jan T. "Triage and Treatment of Radiation-Injured Mass Casualties." http://www.afrri.usuhs.mil. 1989. Accessed.

DuPont, Robert L.; DuPont-Spencer, Elizabeth; DuPont, Caroline M. "Terrorism: Anxiety on a Global Scale." http://www.acsh.org. 2002. Accessed.

"Fact Sheet: Proposed Protective Action Guides for Radiological Dispersion and Improvised Nuclear Devices." http://www.dhs.gov. 2006. Accessed.

Franzius, Enno. History of the Order of the Assassins. Funk and Wagnalls. New York, 1969.

"The Furor Over Fission: The Pros and Cons of Nuclear Power and Trying to Cope with Nuclear Fear." http://www.pbs.org. 1996. Accessed.

González, Abel J. "Timely Action." IAEA Bulletin. http://www.iae.org. 1999. Accessed.

"HHS Public Health Emergency Medical Countermeasure Enterprise, Implementation Plan for Chemical, Biological, Radiological and Nuclear Threats." http://www.hhs.gov. 2007. Accessed.

International Atomic Energy Agency. "Categorization of Radiation Sources." http://www-pub.iaea.org. 2001. Accessed.

Luckett, Larry W.; Vesper, Bruce. "Radiological Considerations in Medical Operations." http://www.afrri.usuhs.mil. 1989. Accessed.

Mallad, Sandhya. "Weapons of Mass Destruction: Chemical, Biological, Radiological and Nuclear (CBRN)." http://www.au.af.mil. 2008. Accessed.

Masters, Donald C. "How to Protect the U.S. Homeland against the Threat of Nuclear and Radiological Terrorism." http://www.hlsia.org. 2008. Accessed.

Medical Preparedness and Response Sub-Group. Department of Homeland Security, Working Group on Radiological Dispersal Device (RDD) Preparedness. http://www1.va.gov. 2003. Accessed.

Mickley, Andrew G. "Psychological Factors in Nuclear Warfare." http://www.afrri.usuhs.mil. 1989. Accessed.

Military Medical Operations, Armed Forces Radiobiology Research Institute. "Medical Management of Radiological Casualties." http://www.afrri.usuhs.mil. 2003. Accessed.

Monsters and Critics. "Experts Rule Out Radioactivity of Meteorite in Peru." http://www.monstersandcritics.com. 2007. Accessed.

Mood, Linda. "Joint Requirements Office for Chemical, Biological, Radiological, and Nuclear Defense." http://www.dtic.mil. 2004. Accessed.

National Institutes of Health. "What We Need to Know About Radiation." http://www.nih.gov. 2000. Accessed.

"NIH Strategic Plan and Research Agenda for Medical Countermeasures Against Radiological and Nuclear Threats." http://www3.niaid.nih.gov. 2005. Accessed.

"Nuclear Reaction: Why Do Americans Fear Nuclear Power?" Frontline show #1511, airdate April 22, 1997; produced and directed by Jon Palfreman; correspondent Richard Rhodes. http://www.pbs.org/wgbh/pages/frontline/reaction/etc/script.html.

OECD Nuclear Energy Agency. *Beneficial Uses and Production of Isotopes: 2000 Update*. 2001.

Peña, Charles. "Smoking Guns, Mushroom Clouds and Fog: Nuclear Fear Factor." http://www.counterpunch.org. 2007. Accessed.

Radiation Basics. http://web.ead/anl.gov/docs/Radiation_Basics.PDF. Argonne National Laboratory, 12/6/99.

Radiochemistry Society Website. http://www.radiochemistry.org. Accessed.

Rennie, Gabriele. "Nuclear Energy to Go." *Science and Technology*. http://www.llnl.gov. 2004. Accessed.

Rennie, Gabriele. "Radiation Detection on the Front Lines." http://www.llnl.gov. 2004. Accessed.

Rockwell, Theodore. "What's Wrong with Being Cautious?" *Nuclear News*, **40**(7): 28–32, June 1997.

Shanker, Thom; McCarthy, Rory. "Nuclear Fear: 'Death of the Indian Subcontinent.'" http://www.smh.com.au. 2002. Accessed.

"Statement of John A. Gordon, Under Secretary of Energy and Administrator for Nuclear Security, National Nuclear Security Administration, U.S. Department of Energy." http://fas.org. 2002. Accessed.

"Strengthening Long-Term Nuclear Security." The National Academies Press, 2005.

Tompkin, Andrew J. "Control and Disposition of Sealed Sources: Relative to a Campus Setting." http://osrp.lanl.gov. 2003. Accessed.

Traynor, Ian. "Blueprint for Nuclear Warhead Found on Smugglers' Computers." http://www.guardian.co.uk. 2008. Accessed.

Waltar, Alan E. "A Day with the Atom . . . Living with Zest!" http://nuclear.tamu.edu. Accessed.

Weart, Spencer R. "Nuclear Fear: A History of Images." Harvard University Press, 1998.

INDEX

*Radiation Safety: Protection and Management for Homeland Security and Emergency
Response.* By L. A. Burchfield
Copyright © 2009 John Wiley & Sons, Inc.